Simulation in Otolaryngology

Editor

SONYA MALEKZADEH

OTOLARYNGOLOGIC CLINICS OF NORTH AMERICA

www.oto.theclinics.com

Consulting Editor
SUJANA S. CHANDRASEKHAR

October 2017 • Volume 50 • Number 5

ELSEVIER

1600 John F. Kennedy Boulevard ● Suite 1800 ● Philadelphia, Pennsylvania, 19103-2899

http://www.oto.theclinics.com

OTOLARYNGOLOGIC CLINICS OF NORTH AMERICA Volume 50, Number 5
October 2017 ISSN 0030-6665, ISBN-13: 978-0-323-54676-8

Editor: Jessica McCool
Developmental Editor: Alison Swety

Otolaryngologic Clinics of North America (ISSN 0030-6665) is published bimonthly by Elsevier, Inc., 360 Park Avenue South, New York, NY 10010-1710. Months of issue are February, April, June, August, October, and December. Business and Editorial Offices: 1600 John F. Kennedy Blvd., Suite 1800, Philadelphia, PA 19103-2899. Customer Service Office: 6277 Sea Harbor Drive, Orlando, FL 32887-4800. Periodicals postage paid at New York, NY and additional mailing offices. Subscription prices are $381.00 per year (US individuals), $803.00 per year (US institutions), $100.00 per year (US student/resident), $500.00 per year (Canadian individuals), $1017.00 per year (Canadian institutions), $556.00 per year (international individuals), $1017.00 per year (international institutions), $270.00 per year (international & Canadian student/resident). Foreign air speed delivery is included in all *Clinics*' subscription prices. All prices are subject to change without notice. **POSTMASTER:** Send address changes to *Otolaryngologic Clinics of North America*, Elsevier Health Sciences Division, Subscription Customer Service, 3251 Riverport Lane, Maryland Heights, MO 63043. **Telephone: 1-800-654-2452 (U.S. and Canada); 314-447-8871 (outside U.S. and Canada). Fax: 314-447-8029. E-mail: journalscustomerservice-usa@elsevier.com (for print support); journalsonlinesupport-usa@elsevier.com (for online support).**

Reprints. For copies of 100 or more of articles in this publication, please contact the Commercial Reprints Department, Elsevier Inc., 360 Park Avenue South, New York, NY 10010-1710. Tel.: 212-633-3874; Fax: 212-633-3820; E-mail: reprints@elsevier.com.

Otolaryngologic Clinics of North America is also published in Spanish by McGraw-Hill Interamericana Editores S.A., P.O. Box 5-237, 06500 Mexico D.F., Mexico.

Otolaryngologic Clinics of North America is covered in *MEDLINE/PubMed (Index Medicus), Current Contents/Clinical Medicine, Excerpta Medica, BIOSIS, Science Citation Index,* and *ISI/BIOMED.*

PROGRAM OBJECTIVE

The goal of the *Otolaryngologic Clinics of North America* is to provide information on the latest trends in patient management, the newest advances; and provide a sound basis for choosing treatment options in the field of otolaryngology.

LEARNING OBJECTIVES

Upon completion of this activity, participants will be able to:
1. Review updates in virtual reality simulation in otolaryngology.
2. Discuss the economics and applications of surgical simulation in otolaryngology.
3. Recognize the use of simulation in the assessment of skills in otolaryngology.

ACCREDITATION

The Elsevier Office of Continuing Medical Education (EOCME) is accredited by the Accreditation Council for Continuing Medical Education (ACCME) to provide continuing medical education for physicians.

The EOCME designates this enduring material for a maximum of 15 *AMA PRA Category 1 Credit*(s)™. Physicians should claim only the credit commensurate with the extent of their participation in the activity.

All other healthcare professionals requesting continuing education credit for this enduring material will be issued a certificate of participation.

DISCLOSURE OF CONFLICTS OF INTEREST

The EOCME assesses conflict of interest with its instructors, faculty, planners, and other individuals who are in a position to control the content of CME activities. All relevant conflicts of interest that are identified are thoroughly vetted by EOCME for fair balance, scientific objectivity, and patient care recommendations. EOCME is committed to providing its learners with CME activities that promote improvements or quality in healthcare and not a specific proprietary business or a commercial interest.

The planning committee, staff, authors and editors listed below have identified no financial relationships or relationships to products or devices they or their spouse/life partner have with commercial interest related to the content of this CME activity:

Lacey K. Adkins, MD; Steven Arild Wuyts Andersen, MD, PhD; Nasir I. Bhatti, MBBS, MD, FRCS; Sarah N. Bowe, MD; James A. Burns, MD, FACS; Sujana S. Chandrasekhar, MD; Seth Dailey, MD; Ellen S. Deutsch, MD, MS; Anjali Fortna; Marvin P. Fried, MD; Kevin Fung, MD; Marc Gibber, MD; Luv Javia, MD; Kaalan Johnson, MD; James A. Kearney, MD; Adam M. Klein, MD, FACS; Andrew Y. Lee, MD; Sonya Malekzadeh, MD; Kelly Michele Malloy, MD, FACS; Jessica McCool; Charles M. Myer IV, MD; Liana Puscas, MD, MHS, MA; Mads Sølvsten Sørensen, MD, DMSc; Maya G. Sardesai, MD, MEd; Carl H. Snyderman, MD, MBA; Jeyanthi Surendrakumar; Alison Swety; Kyle K. VanKoevering, MD; Mark S. Volk, MD, DMD; Katie Widmeier; David H. Yeh, MD.

The planning committee, staff, authors and editors listed below have identified financial relationships or relationships to products or devices they or their spouse/life partner have with commercial interest related to the content of this CME activity:

Noel Jabbour, MD, MS receives royalties/patents from Otologic Skills Simulator and Microsurgical Skills Simulator.
Gregory J. Wiet, MBS, MD has stock ownership in, and an employment affiliation with, Oracle.

UNAPPROVED/OFF-LABEL USE DISCLOSURE

The EOCME requires CME faculty to disclose to the participants:
1. When products or procedures being discussed are off-label, unlabelled, experimental, and/or investigational (not US Food and Drug Administration [FDA] approved); and
2. Any limitations on the information presented, such as data that are preliminary or that represent ongoing research, interim analyses, and/or unsupported opinions. Faculty may discuss information about pharmaceutical agents that is outside of FDA-approved labelling. This information is intended solely for CME and is not intended to promote off-label use of these medications. If you have any questions, contact the medical affairs department of the manufacturer for the most recent prescribing information.

TO ENROLL

To enroll in the *Otolaryngologic Clinics of North America* Continuing Medical Education program, call customer service at 1-800-654-2452 or sign up online at http://www.theclinics.com/home/cme. The CME program is available to subscribers for an additional annual fee of USD 260.

METHOD OF PARTICIPATION

In order to claim credit, participants must complete the following:

1. Complete enrolment as indicated above.
2. Read the activity.
3. Complete the CME Test and Evaluation. Participants must achieve a score of 70% on the test. All CME Tests and Evaluations must be completed online.

CME INQUIRIES/SPECIAL NEEDS

For all CME inquiries or special needs, please contact elsevierCME@elsevier.com.

Contributors

CONSULTING EDITOR

SUJANA S. CHANDRASEKHAR, MD
Director, New York Otology, Clinical Professor, Department of Otolaryngology–Head and Neck Surgery, Hofstra-Northwell School of Medicine, Clinical Associate Professor, Department of Otolaryngology–Head and Neck Surgery, Icahn School of Medicine at Mount Sinai, New York, New York, USA

EDITOR

SONYA MALEKZADEH, MD
Professor, Department of Otolaryngology–Head and Neck Surgery, MedStar Georgetown University Hospital, Washington, DC, USA

AUTHORS

LACEY K. ADKINS, MD
Clinical Fellow, Center for Laryngeal Surgery and Voice Rehabilitation, Massachusetts General Hospital, Boston, Massachusetts, USA

STEVEN ARILD WUYTS ANDERSEN, MD, PhD
Department of Otorhinolaryngology–Head and Neck Surgery, Copenhagen Academy for Medical Education and Simulation, The Simulation Centre, Rigshospitalet, Copenhagen, Denmark

NASIR I. BHATTI, MBBS, MD
Director, Johns Hopkins Percutaneous Trach Service, Associate Professor, Otolaryngology–Head and Neck Surgery, Joint Appointment in Anesthesiology Critical Care Medicine, Baltimore, Maryland, USA

SARAH N. BOWE, MD
Pediatric Otolaryngology Fellow, Department of Otolaryngology–Head and Neck Surgery, Massachusetts Eye and Ear, Boston, Massachusetts, USA

JAMES A. BURNS, MD, FACS
Associate Professor of Surgery, Center for Laryngeal Surgery and Voice Rehabilitation, Massachusetts General Hospital, Boston, Massachusetts, USA

SETH DAILEY, MD
Associate Professor, Division of Otolaryngology, Department of Surgery, University of Wisconsin School of Medicine and Public Health, Madison, Wisconsin, USA

ELLEN S. DEUTSCH, MD, MS
Adjunct Associate Professor and Senior Scientist, Department of Anesthesiology and Critical Care Medicine, Children's Hospital of Philadelphia, Perelman School of Medicine at the University of Pennsylvania, Philadelphia, Pennsylvania, USA; Medical Director, Pennsylvania Patient Safety Authority, Harrisburg, Pennsylvania, USA; ECRI Institute, Plymouth Meeting, Pennsylvania, USA

MARVIN P. FRIED, MD
Chairman and Professor, Department of Otorhinolaryngology–Head and Neck Surgery, Montefiore Medical Center, Albert Einstein College of Medicine, Bronx, New York, USA

KEVIN FUNG, MD
Professor, Department of Otolaryngology–Head and Neck Surgery, London Health Sciences Centre, Victoria Hospital, London, Ontario, Canada

MARC GIBBER, MD
Assistant Professor, Department of Otorhinolaryngology–Head and Neck Surgery, Montefiore Medical Center, Albert Einstein College of Medicine, Bronx, New York, USA

NOEL JABBOUR, MD, MS
Assistant Professor, Division of Pediatric Otolaryngology, Children's Hospital of Pittsburgh of UPMC, Assistant Professor, Department of Otolaryngology, University of Pittsburgh School of Medicine, Pittsburgh, Pennsylvania, USA

LUV JAVIA, MD
Attending Otolaryngologist, Cochlear Implant Program, Center for Pediatric Airway Disorders, Children's Hospital of Philadelphia, Assistant Professor, Department of Clinical Otorhinolaryngology–Head and Neck Surgery, Perelman School of Medicine at the University of Pennsylvania, Philadelphia, Pennsylvania, USA

KAALAN JOHNSON, MD
Assistant Professor, Division of Otolaryngology, Head and Neck Surgery, Seattle Children's Hospital, Seattle, Washington, USA

JAMES A. KEARNEY, MD
Section Chief, Otolaryngology, Pennsylvania Hospital, University of Pennsylvania Health System, Associate Professor, Department of Clinical Otorhinolaryngology–Head and Neck Surgery, Perelman School of Medicine at the University of Pennsylvania, Philadelphia, Pennsylvania, USA

ADAM M. KLEIN, MD, FACS
Associate Professor, Department of Otolaryngology–Head and Neck Surgery, Director, Emory Voice Center, Emory University School of Medicine, Atlanta, Georgia, USA

ANDREW Y. LEE, MD
Department of Otorhinolaryngology–Head and Neck Surgery, Montefiore Medical Center, Albert Einstein College of Medicine, Bronx, New York, USA

SONYA MALEKZADEH, MD
Professor, Department of Otolaryngology–Head and Neck Surgery, MedStar Georgetown University Hospital, Washington, DC, USA

KELLY MICHELE MALLOY, MD, FACS
Associate Professor, Division of Head and Neck Oncology, Department of Otolaryngology–Head and Neck Surgery, University of Michigan, Ann Arbor, Michigan, USA

CHARLES M. MYER IV, MD
Assistant Professor, Division of Pediatric Otolaryngology, Department of Otolaryngology–Head and Neck Surgery, Cincinnati Children's Hospital Medical Center, University of Cincinnati College of Medicine, Cincinnati, Ohio, USA

LIANA PUSCAS, MD, MHS, MA
Associate Professor, Division of Head and Neck Surgery and Communication Sciences, Duke University Medical Center, Durham, North Carolina, USA

MAYA G. SARDESAI, MD, MEd
Associate Professor, Otolaryngology–Head and Neck Surgery, University of Washington, Seattle, Washington, USA

CARL H. SNYDERMAN, MD, MBA
Professor, Departments of Otolaryngology and Neurological Surgery, Center for Cranial Base Surgery, The Eye & Ear Institute, University of Pittsburgh School of Medicine, Pittsburgh, Pennsylvania, USA

MADS SØLVSTEN SØRENSEN, MD, DMSc
Department of Otorhinolaryngology–Head and Neck Surgery, Rigshospitalet, Copenhagen, Denmark

KYLE K. VANKOEVERING, MD
Fellow, Anterior Cranial Base Surgery, Department of Otolaryngology–Head and Neck Surgery, The Ohio State University Wexner Medical Center, Columbus, Ohio, USA

MARK S. VOLK, MD, DMD
Associate Attending, Department of Otolaryngology and Communication Disorders, Associate Clinical Director, Otolaryngology Programs, Simulator Program, Boston Children's Hospital, Assistant Professor, Department of Otolaryngology, Harvard Medical School, Boston, Massachusetts, USA

GREGORY J. WIET, MBS, MD
Professor, Departments of Otolaryngology, Pediatrics, and Biomedical Informatics, Nationwide Children's Hospital, The Ohio State University, Columbus, Ohio, USA

DAVID H. YEH, MD
Clinical Fellow, Department of Otolaryngology–Head and Neck Surgery, London Health Sciences Centre, Victoria Hospital, London, Ontario, Canada

Contents

during otolaryngology residency training. Simulators are useful for developing laryngeal and airway surgery skills ultimately evaluated in a competency-based manner.

Simulation is an emerging and viable means to increase pediatric airway surgical training. A variety of simulators currently exist that may be used or modified for laryngoscopy, bronchoscopy, and endoscopic intervention, although anatomic realism and utility for complex procedures are limited. There is a need for further development of improved endoscopic and anatomic models. Innovative techniques are enabling small-scale manufacturing of generalizable and patient-specific simulators. The high acuity of the pediatric airway patient makes the use of simulation an attractive modality for training, competency maintenance, and patient safety quality-improvement studies.

This article presents a summary of the current simulation training for otologic skills. There is a wide variety of educational approaches, assessment tools, and simulators in use, including simple low-cost task trainers to complex computer-based virtual reality systems. A systematic approach to otologic skills training using adult learning theory concepts, such as repeated and distributed practice, self-directed learning, and mastery learning, is necessary for these educational interventions to be effective. Future directions include development of measures of performance to assess efficacy of simulation training interventions and, for complex procedures, improvement in fidelity based on educational goals.

Simulation is rapidly expanding across medicine as a valuable component of trainee education. For procedural simulation, development of low-cost simulators that allow a realistic, haptic experience for learners to practice maneuvers while appreciating anatomy has become highly valuable. Otolaryngology has seen significant advancements in development of improved, specialty-specific simulators with the expansion of 3-dimensional (3D) printing. This article highlights the fundamental components of 3D printing and the multitude of subspecialty simulators that have been developed with the assistance of 3D printing. It briefly discusses important considerations such as cost, fidelity, and validation where available in the literature.

Evaluation of surgical skills and competency are important aspects of the medical education process. Measurable and reproducible methods of assessment with objective feedback are essential components of surgical training. Objective Structured Assessment of Technical Skills (OSATS) is widely used across the medical specialties, and otolaryngology-specific tools have been developed and validated for sinus and mastoid surgery. Although assessment of surgical skills can be time-consuming and requires human and financial resources, new evaluation methods and emerging technology may alleviate these barriers while also improving data collection practices.

American health care is facing an epidemic of medical errors. A major cause of these errors is poor teamwork. Crisis resource management (CRM) is a set of teamwork principles derived from the airline industry. Medical simulation is an educational tool that affords health care providers a means of improving teamwork by learning and practicing CRM. This chapter discusses: 1) The case for teaching team training. 2) Review the principles of medical simulation as it pertains to team training. 3) Provide practical guidelines for using medical simulation in Otolaryngology education. 4) Discuss current evidence of the efficacy of medical simulation.

Successful simulation requires effective facilitation and debriefing to achieve educational goals. Simulation educational methods are diverse, ranging from partial task training to complicated, interdisciplinary team training. Various debriefing models have emerged based on method of instruction, learner experience, time and equipment capability, and physical facilities. The general structure of most debriefing sessions focuses on participant reactions, followed by analysis, and ending with a discussion of lessons learned. Two leading debriefing models, the Structured and Supported Debriefing Model and the Debriefing with Good Judgment Model, are described in further detail.

Simulation-based boot camps are growing in popularity and are effective in onboarding novice residents with new knowledge, skills, and behaviors. These intensive and immersive courses may be used to train residents and allied health professionals in specific procedures, teamwork, and management of rare clinical scenarios. A needs assessment of learners determines the course curriculum. Boot camps are designed to encourage active and hands-on participation with deliberate practice and immediate feedback. As surgical education shifts toward competency-based medical education, there may be an even greater role for simulation-based boot camps as a training and assessment tool.

Attempts to understand and improve health care delivery often focus on the characteristics of the patient and the characteristics of the health care providers, but larger systems surround and integrate with patients and providers. Components of health care delivery systems can support or interfere with efforts to provide optimal health care. Simulation in situ, involving real teams participating in simulations in real care settings, can be used to identify latent safety threats and improve the work environment while simultaneously supporting participant learning. Thoughtful planning and skilled debriefing are essential.

There are massive hidden costs in the current paradigm of surgical training related to increased operative times for procedures with resident involvement and costs of medical errors. Shifting procedural training outside of the operating room through use of simulation has the potential to improve patient safety, minimize learning time to achieve competency, and increase operative efficiency. Investment in surgical simulation has the potential to reduce costs to health care systems through improved operating room efficiency and reduction of medical errors. This article explores the economic costs related to surgical training in otolaryngology and the value of investment in surgical simulation.

OTOLARYNGOLOGIC CLINICS OF NORTH AMERICA

RELATED INTEREST

Oral and Maxillofacial Clinics of North America
May 2017 (Vol. 29, Issue 2)
Patient Safety
David W. Todd and Jeffrey D. Bennett, *Editors*
Available at: http://www.oralmaxsurgery.theclinics.com/

THE CLINICS ARE AVAILABLE ONLINE!
Access your subscription at:
www.theclinics.com

Foreword

See One, Do One, Teach One: No More

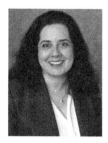

Sujana S. Chandrasekhar, MD
Consulting Editor

Anatomic dissection prior to examining and treating a living person dates back to Alexandria, Greece in the third century BC.[1] For Otolaryngologist-Head and Neck Surgeons, anatomic dissections, the original "simulators," have served to prepare them for open approaches to the face, head, and neck, for temporal bone surgery, and for paranasal sinus procedures. But, as with diagnostic and surgical methods and tools, simulation tools and techniques have evolved, most rapidly over the past several years.

In this issue of *Otolaryngologic Clinics of North America*, Dr Malekzadeh has compiled a thoughtful and thorough review of the state-of-the-art in simulation. The authors of each article share their perspectives on improved education in the field as well as using simulation and technology to better assess trainees' surgical skills and competency, and for enhancing team performance. The reader who can benefit from this Otolaryngologic Clinics of North America issue ranges from trainee to senior otolaryngologist and those in academic to private practice. This issue will be of interest to those who are responsible for oversight of medical student and otolaryngology resident/fellow education and anyone who is committed to continuing education and self-improvement.

Given the scarcity, cost, and relative unavailability of "original" simulators of cadaveric human tissue, the lifelong learner of Otolaryngology should become familiar with the newer physical models and virtual reality simulators that are available during training and beyond. The surgeon who has become familiar with endonasal and other rhinologic approaches, with airway management in adults and children, and with simple to complex otologic procedures with near-natural haptic feedback, all via simulation carried out in a nonstressful setting where repeated practice is possible, will be a better-prepared surgeon when operating in the real setting. I, personally, have drilled out a mastoid on a 3D printed temporal bone; the realism is astonishing.

Otolaryngol Clin N Am 50 (2017) xv–xvi
http://dx.doi.org/10.1016/j.otc.2017.07.002
0030-6665/17/© 2017 Published by Elsevier Inc.

oto.theclinics.com

Residents in Otolaryngology have much to learn in a shortened time period. Using simulation the way it is described in the Boot Camp article helps make the initial ramp-up significantly easier, more efficient, and less frightening. That first real peritonsillar abscess will be identified and drained more effectively by someone who has already completed a simulation scenario complete with popping open the "peritonsillar space" full of gelatin goo in their low-cost trainer. Similar scenarios are used to teach Advanced Cardiac Life Support to all physicians; the scenarios on emergency Otolaryngology presentations take the panic and guesswork out of a real-life situation.

All of this enhances patient care and health care team performance. That first month of residency should no longer be a period of trepidation for trainee, supervisor, or patient. Residents trained on simulators can function quasi-independently and on teams with confidence. Educators now have these validated tools by which to assess skills and competency. Future partners and employers can be secure regarding their new colleagues, and patient care systems can become more efficient.

Surgical simulation has come a long way from just late nights in the dissection laboratory. I congratulate Dr Malekzadeh as guest editor and all the authors who have contributed their knowledge and ideas to this issue of *Otolaryngologic Clinics of North America*, and I hope you, the reader, enjoy it.

Sujana S. Chandrasekhar, MD
Director
New York Otology
Clinical Professor
Department of Otolaryngology–Head and Neck Surgery
Hofstra-Northwell School of Medicine
Clinical Associate Professor
Department of Otolaryngology–Head and Neck Surgery
Icahn School of Medicine at Mount Sinai
1421 Third Avenue, 4th Floor
New York, NY 10028, USA

E-mail address:
ssc@nyotology.com

REFERENCE

1. Ghosh SK. Human cadaveric dissection: a historical account from ancient Greece to the modern era. Anat Cell Biol 2015;48(3):153–69. http://dx.doi.org/10.5115/acb.2015.48.3.153.

Preface

Simulation in Otolaryngology

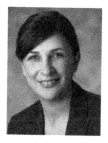

Sonya Malekzadeh, MD
Editor

At present, simulation is widely accepted as a means of providing surgical education outside of the clinical environment. Recent advances in simulation technology and medical education reform coupled with political and societal demands have provided the impetus toward the exponential growth of this field. Research in this area supports the use of simulation to train and assess individuals in both psychomotor and team-based skills. Further benefits include translation of these improved skills to patient care practices with better patient outcomes and reduced health care costs.

This issue of *Otolaryngologic Clinics of North America* introduces into the literature a collection of work dedicated to simulation in otolaryngology. The history of medical simulation stretches back over centuries, and otolaryngologists have been longtime users of simulation: the tradition of training on cadaveric temporal bones and managing complex airway situations on manikins are integral parts of our specialty. As illustrated by the quantity and quality of material in this issue, otolaryngologists are furthering the field of simulation via innovative simulators and curricular development while promoting the importance of team-based and interprofessional approaches to learning and health care. The authors were chosen because of their published expertise in each subject area and because of their national reputation as leaders in simulation. I am deeply appreciative of their time and efforts in developing this comprehensive view of simulation in otolaryngology that will serve as an

Otolaryngol Clin N Am 50 (2017) xvii–xviii
http://dx.doi.org/10.1016/j.otc.2017.07.001
0030-6665/17/© 2017 Published by Elsevier Inc.

oto.theclinics.com

invaluable reference for all involved in the training and education of future otolaryngologists.

Sonya Malekzadeh, MD
Department of Otolaryngology–Head and Neck Surgery
MedStar Georgetown University Hospital
3800 Reservoir Road, NW
1 Gorman
Washington, DC 20007, USA

E-mail address:
malekzas@georgetown.edu

Physical Models and Virtual Reality Simulators in Otolaryngology

Luv Javia, MD[a],*, Maya G. Sardesai, MD, MEd[b]

KEYWORDS

- Physical simulator • Virtual reality • Simulators • Medical education
- Otolaryngology

KEY POINTS

- Otolaryngology, like other surgical disciplines, is increasingly relying on simulators for educating its trainees.
- Physical simulators are models with which the learner physically interacts to improve knowledge and skills.
- Virtual-reality simulators allow the learner to interact with an environment that is computer generated to enhance knowledge and skills.
- The types of simulators available in otolaryngology are as diverse as are the subspecialties, and new simulators are continually being developed.

Over the years, as the role of simulation in medical education has become more established, otolaryngologists have developed a plethora of simulators. Modern training relies increasingly on simulation in some form to teach everything from basic suturing to complex multidisciplinary patient care scenarios. Simulators allow for teaching trainees in a low-stress environment that does not result in real patient morbidity and mortality, and allows for pauses, reflection, and discussion.

Simulators in otolaryngology mimic the variety of surgical techniques and environments present in this surgical subspecialty. There is also a range of simulators including physical and virtual-reality simulators. Physical simulators are models with which the operator can physically interact. In contrast, virtual-reality simulators allow the operator to interact with an environment that is generated by a computer. This

Disclosure Statement: Neither author has any relevant disclosures.
[a] Children's Hospital of Philadelphia, 3401 Civic Center Boulevard, 1 Wood Building, Philadelphia, PA 19104, USA; [b] Harborview Medical Center, Box 359894, 325 Ninth Avenue, Seattle, WA 98104, USA
* Corresponding author.
E-mail address: javia@email.chop.edu

Otolaryngol Clin N Am 50 (2017) 875–891
http://dx.doi.org/10.1016/j.otc.2017.05.001
0030-6665/17/© 2017 Elsevier Inc. All rights reserved.

oto.theclinics.com

article presents some of the most studied and useful physical and virtual-reality simulators in otolaryngology.

PHYSICAL SIMULATORS

Physical simulators are models that can be as specific as a body part, such as a larynx or temporal bone; but it can also involve a model of an entire human being. Total body simulators, such as SimMan, SimNewB, or SimBaby (Laerdal, Stavanger, Norway), are used in complex patient scenarios to train residents how to deal with critical situations that may not be encountered as often. Physical models can be directly palpated, manipulated, incised, and modified. Examples of physical models include task trainers or simulation mannequins.

Among the strengths of physical simulators is that they are low cost, easy to assemble, and easy to maintain. Many simulators described in the literature are constructed from easily available materials. This makes it readily accessible to training programs and trainees. Physical simulators can also be high tech, involving feedback and electronics that augment the simulation experience. Physical simulators are used in the various subspecialties of otolaryngology.

Airway and Laryngeal Physical Simulators

Laryngeal and airway physical simulators are some of the most commonly used simulators, and can appeal to audiences beyond otolaryngology (**Table 1**). There are several airway simulators based on using biologic tissues, such as porcine or ovine, for performing microlaryngoscopy and bronchoscopy even with foreign body removal.[1,2]

Nonbiologic physical models to train basic intubation skills have been used for some time,[3] and current models include the complexity of varying anatomy, including neonatal, pediatric, and adult simulators.[4–6] There are even models for the premature neonate. Laerdal is one such company that supplies a variety of commonly used physical simulators. At a bootcamp held at our institution, airway simulators have been used to teach airway skills, such as intubation and airway foreign body removal.[1] Mannequins with a head and lower airways are used to teach intubation to younger residents and bronchoscopy skills. Junior residents can practice retrieving airway foreign bodies placed by attending surgeons who teach at these skills workstations. Additional modifications can include using a high-fidelity mannequin that can have vital signs presented on a screen. These vital signs can be manipulated to simulate such factors as hypoxemia or recovery depending on how the resident is able to intervene with the staged simulation scenario. A smoke machine has also been used to simulate a surgical drape fire, such as may be encountered if the resident does not correctly pay attention to placement of bronchoscopic equipment on operative drapes, or to simulate an airway fire.

Full-body high-fidelity mannequin can also be useful in setting up complex patient scenarios. High-fidelity elements that increase realism in simulation can include chest wall motion (even single-sided chest wall movement to simulate bronchial intubation or foreign body), eye blinking, ability for a confederate to speak remotely on the mannequin's behalf, programmable vital signs, altered head and neck mobility, reduced mouth and glottic opening, increased tongue volume, and pharyngeal obstruction. Full-body mannequins are used in airway scenarios, such as false passage with tracheostomy, pneumothorax requiring needle decompression, and airway foreign body or hemorrhage requiring bronchoscopy. There are other nonairway scenarios, such as intraoperative air embolism and surgical fire. The high-fidelity mannequin

Table 1
Airway and laryngeal simulators

Simulator	Type	Authors	Notes
Animal airway simulator	Physical	Deutsch et al,[1] 2009; Ianacone et al,[2] 2016	Porcine and ovine models for microlaryngoscopy and bronchoscopy
Laerdal adult mannequin	Physical	Howells et al,[3] 1973	Adult mannequin used for endotracheal intubation
SimMan	Physical	Hesselfeldt et al,[4] 2005	SimMan full-scale simulator
SimBaby	Physical	Schebesta et al,[5] 2011	SimBaby high-fidelity simulator
Neonatal airway simulators	Physical	Sawyer et al,[6] 2016	Evaluation of eight different neonatal airway simulators
Intubation and airway foreign body removal	Physical	Deutsch et al,[1] 2009	Describe various simulators for airway endoscopy
Nasolaryngoscopy	Physical	Smith et al,[8] 2014	Mannequin-based nasolaryngoscopy training
Cadaveric larynges	Physical	Amin et al,[9] 2007	Vocal fold injection
Porcine larynges	Physical	Dedmon et al,[10] 2015	Vocal fold augmentation, excision of a simulated vocal fold nodule, and excision of a simulated vocal fold keratosis
Porcine larynges	Physical	Awad et al,[11] 2015	Vocal fold biopsy, vocal fold medialization injection, submucosal flap elevation, posterior cordotomy
Porcine larynges in mannequin	Physical	Nixon et al,[12] 2012	Resection of laryngeal lesions
Synthetic vocal fold module inserted into mannequin	Physical	Fleming et al,[13] 2012	Laryngoscopy and resection of polypoid lesion
Synthetic multilayered vocal folds	Physical	Contag et al,[14] 2009	Resection of superficial vocal fold lesion
Modular laryngeal cartridges	Physical	Holliday et al,[15] 2015	Laryngeal cartridges made from rubber bands enclosed in plastic wrap within polyvinyl chloride pipe; papilloma debulking, subepithelial and epithelial lesion excision
Transcervical laryngeal injection trainer	Physical	Cabrera-Muffly et al,[16] 2016	Transcervical injection simulator made from toilet paper tube, thin balloon, and other easily found materials
Transcervical laryngeal injection trainer	Physical	Ainsworth et al,[17] 2014	3D-printed laryngotracheal framework with tactile and auditory feedback

(continued on next page)

Table 1 (continued)			
Simulator	Type	Authors	Notes
Endoscopic psychomotor skills trainer	Physical	Ross et al,[18] 2015	3D-printed model with electromagnetic tracking system and LED lights; endoscopic skills trainer
Bronchoscopy	Virtual reality	Rowe & Cohen,[60] 2002; Deutsch et al,[1] 2009	AccuTouch flexible bronchoscopy simulator
Bronchoscopy	Virtual reality	Pastis et al,[58] 2014	Simbionix bronchoscopy simulator
Bronchoscopy	Virtual reality	Vaidyanath et al,[59] 2013	ORSIM bronchoscopy simulator
Bronchoscopy simulator	Virtual reality	http://www.thoracic-anesthesia.com/	Online bronchoscopy simulator

Abbreviation: 3D, three-dimensional.

have been set up in mock operating rooms with attending surgeons acting as confederates to run scenarios in which an individual resident or groups of residents are assigned different roles. These full-body mannequins can also be modified to suit one's needs. For example, we have placed puffed rice cereal under simulated skin to imitate subcutaneous emphysema and crepitus. Immersion in such a situation is a powerful experience for residents to see how they would perform in emergent situations.

Other simulators are partial body simulators or task trainers that can be used for teaching intubation, bronchoscopy, or nasolaryngoscopy.[7,8] One advantage of the partial anatomic simulators is their ease of portability; these can easily be taken from one place to another or from one workshop to another.

More recently, a plethora of simulators have been developed by laryngologists. Traditionally, human or porcine larynges served as a platform for performing laryngeal surgeries, such as vocal fold biopsy, vocal fold medialization with an injection, or submucosal vocal fold flap elevation.[9–12] The use of biologic tissues, however, adds the complexities of maintaining facilities for use of these biologic specimens, difficult procurement of specimens, and the difficulty of portability. This has led to the development of nonbiologic physical simulators. Laryngology simulators include custom-produced vocal fold replicas[13]; fabricated laryngeal models with replaceable vocal folds[14]; modular laryngeal cartridges created from rubber bands enclosed in plastic wrap within a polyvinyl chloride pipe[15]; laryngeal injection simulator constructed from toilet paper tube, zip tie, thin balloon, and other easily found objects[16]; three-dimensional (3D) printed laryngotracheal framework[17]; and 3D printed model with an electromagnetic tracking system.[18] Not all physical models necessitate custom manufactured systems. In fact, there are a few ingenious physical models that are more readily constructed.[15,16] Specifically, the Georgetown Laryngeal Model[15] is creative, capable of simulating a wide variety of laryngology surgical procedures on one basic platform. It is used to grasp and cut sutures from the vocal folds, to resect an epithelial lesion, a subepithelial lesion, and laryngeal papillomas. The simplicity and modularity of this model makes it a favorite at our regional bootcamp for otolaryngology residents.

3D printing is being increasingly used to construct custom anatomy and pathology. This ability to produce custom physical models has powerful potential for the future of simulators and simulation (discussed elsewhere in this issue). A group has already constructed a 3D-printed high-fidelity laryngeal framework used with molded arytenoid cartilages and intrinsic laryngeal musculature.[17] The thyroarytenoid muscle, constructed with conductive silicone, allows for real-time feedback of successful needle placement during transcervical vocal fold injection. 3D printing is an area of tremendous growth and potential in the future as access increases at various institutions. 3D printing will also allow for a variety of pathologies to be able to be replicated, so that the learner can encounter different patient scenarios. Additionally, electronics can be imbedded into 3D-printed physical models to add additional elements of realism or feedback. Ross and colleagues[18] created a 3D-printed airway with imbedded LEDs that was used to teach endoscopic psychomotor skills.

Otology Physical Simulators

Otology is perhaps one of the most developed subspecialties in otolaryngology in terms of simulators (**Table 2**). Myringotomy and ear tube placement is a common first surgical procedure for residents. Simple myringotomy and ear tube simulators can help the novice gain exposure to this procedure before performing on real patients. At our institution, most junior residents use a simple physical model to practice this procedure with a microscope before performing on a patient. Physical models constructed from parts, both readily available and inexpensive, have been used in several simulators for myringotomy with ear tube insertion.[19–22] Many are fabricated with syringes that simulate the external auditory canal with disposable gloves used to mimic the tympanic membrane. Construction is easy and these physical simulators can be repeatedly used for multiple attempts. Volsky and colleagues[19] describe a patented model that consists of a canal component, a cartridge component, and a head component. Despite this model's greater fidelity of the auricle and ear canal, a consideration is that this simulator may require purchase of basic units or pieces for use.

Physical simulators for middle ear procedures have also been described. Pettigrew temporal bones were modified to host a middle ear module such that stapedotomy and various other ossiculoplasty procedures could be performed. Unfortunately, to the best of our knowledge, this is not commercially available.[23] Similarly, the middle ear ossicles with adjacent structures, such as tendons, nerves, and ligaments, were 3D printed and loaded in a cartridge by another group.[24] They described using this model to perform a stapedotomy; however, this could also be a valuable and novel platform to perform various middle ear surgeries. Recently, a low-cost microsurgery ear trainer has been described that allows removal of ear canal foreign body, myringotomy tube placement, tympanomeatal flap elevation, myringoplasty, and a middle ear task.[25]

With the increasing popularity of endoscopic ear surgery, there has also been development of simulators for training purposes. The transcanal endoscopic ear surgery simulator is a reusable 3D-printed task trainer in which trainees manipulate rings between pegs in a middle ear chamber accessed by endoscopic equipment through a simulated ear canal.[26] An ovine model has been used to perform endoscopic ear surgery.[27] This model was used to perform canalplasty, middle ear dissection, myringoplasty, and ossiculoplasty.

Physical temporal bone simulators have been developed to teach the central skill of temporal bone drilling to otolaryngology trainees. Traditionally cadaveric temporal bones have been and continue to be the mainstay of teaching drilling. However, these are becoming increasingly more difficult and expensive to obtain. Physical models of temporal bones can be drilled with irrigation and suction. Some are synthetic temporal

Table 2
Otology simulators

Simulator	Type	Authors	Notes
Myringotomy and ear tube insertion	Physical	Volsky et al,[19] 2009	Model designed from three plastic parts
Myringotomy and ear tube insertion	Physical	Malekzadeh et al,[20] 2011	Model constructed from 3-mL syringe, plastic glove, and glove box
Myringotomy and ear tube insertion	Physical	Hong et al,[21] 2014	Model constructed from 3-mL syringe, vinyl glove, and plastic base
Myringotomy and ear tube insertion	Physical	Estomba et al,[22] 2015	Model constructed from 5-mL syringe, latex glove, and wood
Modified Pettigrew temporal bones with middle ear module	Physical	Mills & Lee,[23] 2003	Pettigrew temporal bones modified with middle ear module; stapedectomy and various other ossiculoplasty procedures
3D-printed middle ear module	Physical	Monfared et al,[24] 2012	3D-printed and loaded cartridge; stapedectomy and potential for various other middle ear surgeries
Low-cost microsurgery ear trainer	Physical	Clark et al,[25] 2016	Simulates removal of ear canal foreign body, myringotomy tube placement, tympanomeatal flap elevation, myringoplasty, and a middle ear task
3D-printed transcanal endoscopic ear surgery simulator	Physical	Barber et al,[26] 2016	3D-printed task trainer for transcanal endoscopic ear surgery
Ovine endoscopic ear surgery simulator	Physical	Anschuetz et al,[27] 2016	Ovine model used to perform endoscopic canalplasty, middle ear dissection, myringoplasty, and ossiculoplasty
Pettigrew temporal bones	Physical	Awad et al,[28] 2014	Synthetic temporal bones for drilling
3D-printed temporal bone	Physical	Da Cruz & Francis,[29] 2015	3D-printed temporal bone used for drilling
3D-printed temporal bone	Physical	Mick et al,[30] 2013	Ultra-high-resolution computed tomography images of temporal bone used to construct 3D-printed bone for drilling
3D-printed temporal bone	Physical	Mowry et al,[31] 2015	3D-printed temporal bone used for drilling
3D-printed temporal bone	Physical	Hochman et al,[32] 2015	3D-printed temporal bone used for drilling
3D-printed temporal bone	Physical	Rose et al,[33] 2015	Multicolor, multimaterial 3D-printed temporal bone printed using micro computed tomography data

(continued on next page)

Table 2 *(continued)*			
Simulator	**Type**	**Authors**	**Notes**
Otoscopy	Virtual reality	Lee et al,[62] 2015	OtoSim, model ear and otoscope used to view high-fidelity images of tympanic membrane and middle ear pathology
Myringotomy	Virtual reality	Wheeler et al,[63] 2010	Optical tracker
Myringotomy	Virtual reality	Sowerby et al,[64] 2010; Ho et al,[65] 2012	Haptic feedback
Temporal bone drilling	Virtual reality	Zirkle et al,[66] 2007	VOXEL-MAN surgical simulator
Temporal bone drilling	Virtual reality	Wiet et al,[67] 2002	Ohio State University surgical simulator
Temporal bone drilling	Virtual reality	Sewell et al,[68] 2008	Stanford surgical simulator
Temporal bone drilling	Virtual reality	Zhao et al,[69] 2011	Mediseus surgical simulator

bones that can be purchased, such as the Pettigrew temporal bone.[28] Pettigrew temporal bones provide similar haptic feedback to cadaveric temporal bones, allowing the use of suction and irrigation, possessing important landmarks painted for identification, and containing articulating ossicles. However, Pettigrew temporal bones are thought to have inaccurate facial nerve anatomy in the region of the second genu. Experts agree that using this simulator could improve global transferrable otologic skills, but that facial nerve anatomic concerns should be addressed before recommending this model.

Many have also described 3D-printed temporal bones for drilling purposes.[29–33] The 3D-printed models can be customized, allowing exposure to different pathologic situations. Rose and colleagues[33] created a multicolor, multimaterial 3D-printed temporal bone based on micro computed tomography data that demonstrated face validity. One of the challenges mentioned by the authors is that current 3D printing technology requires a support structure that can inhibit such surgical simulation as cochlear implant insertion. Another concern was cost. As 3D printing technology continues to evolve, the belief is that these issues will be alleviated. Clearly, one of the powers of using 3D printing to create physical simulators is that the possibilities of simulating a myriad of pathologies are endless.

Sinus/Rhinology Physical Simulators

There has also been rapid expansion in the development of physical model task trainers in rhinology (**Table 3**). Sinus surgery is technically challenging and high stakes, as the most commonly litigated field of otolaryngology with among the highest payouts.[34] Historically, human and animal cadavers and live animal models[2,35] have provided the mainstay of ex vivo training, but these are burdensome with respect to cost and storage.

Among the best-described physical models is a low-cost task trainer developed by Malekzadeh and colleagues.[36] It uses a stainless stainless-steel bread pan; unflavored gelatin; eggs; and silicone cardiopulmonary resuscitation mannequin mask (Laerdal,

Table 3
Sinus/rhinology simulators

Simulator	Type	Authors	Notes
Endoscopic rhinology trainer	Physical	Awad et al,[35] 2014	Sheep heads used for endoscopic training
Sinus surgery task trainer	Physical	Malekzadeh et al,[36] 2011	Gelatin-based simulator embedded with various objects and covered with cardiopulmonary resuscitation mask
Seattle sinus simulator	Physical	Harbison et al,[38] 2017	Constructed of silicone, Styrofoam, and silicone mannequin mask
Nasal endoscopy simulator	Virtual reality	Ecke et al,[72] 1998	Head model with graphics workstation
Nasal endoscopy simulator	Virtual reality	Caversaccio et al,[73] 2003; Tolsdorff et al,[74] 2010	With haptic feedback
Endoscopic Sinus Surgery Simulator (ES3)	Virtual reality	Edmond,[71] 2002	Haptic feedback; collects and analyzes performance data; able to give feedback in real time

Wappinger Falls, NY) to recreate a basic nasal cavity, maxillary sinus, and nasopharynx. This model enables trainees to perform such tasks as probing sinus recesses, removing fluid from the maxillary sinus, and targeted injections. Addition of materials, such as suture and plastic beads, teaches grasping and tissue removal tasks. The model was shown to have face, content, and construct validity.[37] At a total cost of less than $5, it is accessible to trainees at all levels. A limitation of this model, however, is that the biologic materials (eggs) are prone to decomposition, which limits the potential for intermittent or just-in-time training.

To address this issue, the Seattle Sinus Simulator was developed. It uses exclusively nonbiologic materials including moldable silicone, Styrofoam, and a silicone mannequin mask.[38] Trainees can perform tasks including endoscopic visualization, suctioning, targeted injections, and "tissue" removal from various locations. In combination with a knowledge-based curriculum, the model has been shown to have face, content, and construct validity, and with an overall cost of less than $15. However, the model does require construction, and may ultimately be prone to wear and tear, which has yet to be quantified.

Miscellaneous Physical Simulators

Several simulators fall outside the described categories, yet are valuable additions to otolaryngologic training (**Table 4**). Junior residents are called on frequently to help gain control over epistaxis. Cadaveric heads have been used to construct a high-fidelity task trainer in which intravenous (IV) tubing is positioned through the posterior cribriform plate and nasal cavity simulating a sphenopalatine artery bleed.[39] An epistaxis physical simulator can be constructed from an old, modified cardiopulmonary resuscitation trainer.[40,41] Red dye fluid running through the IV simulates active bleeding and makes the experience more realistic.

Another common procedure for the junior resident is tonsillectomy. Surprisingly, there is a paucity of reported physical simulators for performing this procedure. However, there are several for ligation of bleeding vessels as may be encountered during tonsillectomy.[42–45]

Table 4
Miscellaneous simulators

Simulator	Type	Authors	Notes
Epistaxis	Physical	Scott et al,[39] 2016	Cadaveric heads with IV tubing to simulate sphenopalatine artery bleed
Epistaxis	Physical	Malekzadeh et al,[41] 2014; Pettineo et al,[40] 2008	Modified cardiopulmonary resuscitation trainer with active bleeding
Ligation of vessels (during tonsillectomy)	Physical	Pearson & Wallace,[42] 1997	Plastic cup and gauze used to construct simulator for ligating vessels
Ligation of vessels (during tonsillectomy)	Physical	Duodu & Lesser,[43] 2013	Intubation mouth model, latex glove, and IV fluid/tubing used to make a simulator for ligating vessels; active bleeding
Ligation of vessels (during tonsillectomy)	Physical	Raja et al,[44] 2008	Skull model and nasal gauze with red food coloring used to make a simulator for ligating vessels
Ligation of vessels (during tonsillectomy)	Physical	Street et al,[45] 2006	Model for ligating vessels constructed from child's shoe and examination gloves
Peritonsillar abscess drainage	Physical	Bunting et al,[46] 2015	Knox gelatin, water balloon, and mannequin head used to create simulator
Peritonsillar abscess drainage	Physical	Scott et al,[47] 2016	Cadaveric head and latex gloves used to create simulator
Peritonsillar abscess drainage	Physical	Taylor & Chang,[48] 2014	Latex moulage of tonsils with latex balloon mounted on polyvinyl chloride pipe
Peritonsillar abscess drainage	Physical	Giblett & Hari,[49] 2016	Silicone tonsil mold with cod liver oil capsule inserted into mannequin head
Suturing and local flap reconstruction	Physical	Janus & Hamilton,[50] 2013	Open-cell foam and elastic foam tape used to simulate skin for suturing and local flap execution
Facial local flap reconstruction	Physical	Gilmour et al,[51] 2012	Model head with layered pigmented latex to simulate various anatomic elements
Facial local flap reconstruction	Physical	Taylor & Chang,[52] 2016	Gelatin prosthetic facial skin simulator used to perform Z-plasty, bilobed, rhomboid, and paramedian forehead flap
Ovine dissection model	Physical	Ianacone et al,[2] 2016	Blepharoplasty, ptosis repair, orbital floor exploration, facial nerve dissection and repair, mandibular plating, tracheotomy, laryngofissure, tracheal resection and laryngectomy

(continued on next page)

Table 4 (continued)			
Simulator	**Type**	**Authors**	**Notes**
Neck dissection	Physical	Griffin et al,[53] 2013	Modified blue phantom central line placement training model
Robotic surgery	Physical	Sperry et al,[54] 2014	Used robotic setup to perform dissections on cadaveric heads
Rigid esophagoscopy	Physical	Allak et al,[55] 2016	Plaster skull, injection mold of esophagus, and force sensors
Da Vinci Skills Simulator	Virtual reality	Walliczek et al,[82] 2016; Walliczek-Dworschak et al,[83] 2017; Zhang & Sumer,[84] 2013	Robotic Skills Simulator
Subtotal/ intracapsular tonsillectomy	Virtual reality	Ruthenbeck et al,[85] 2012	Tonsillectomy simulator with haptic feedback, and visual and auditory cues
Fine-needle aspiration biopsy of thyroid	Virtual reality	Souza et al,[86] 2009	Haptic feedback enabled

Abbreviation: IV, intravenous.

Several physical simulators exist for peritonsillar abscess drainage.[46–49] All are easily constructed: water balloons in gelatin, latex glove filled with vanilla pudding, or even cod liver oil capsules imbedded in silicone tonsil molds. Simulated tonsils with abscesses were inserted into an oral cavity/pharynx either of a cadaveric head, task trainer, or polyvinyl chloride pipe.

Physical simulators can also provide benefit to residents for complex wound closure as seen commonly in facial plastics. At our institution's bootcamp, we use a pig's foot, on which various skin defects are created and reconstructed using a variety of local flaps. This is consistently a popular station with the residents, because it allows them to perform various flaps in a low-stress environment. Other groups have used readily available hospital supplies, such as open-cell foam and elastic foam tape to practice a variety of interrupted suturing maneuvers and constructing and executing local flaps.[50] Others use a polystyrene head with molded latex on top that can then be used to create facial defects and perform flap reconstruction.[51] Likewise, Z-plasty, bilobed, rhomboid, and paramedian forehead flaps can be performed on a low-cost gelatin prosthetic facial skin simulator.[52]

Ianacone and colleagues[2] have reported on ovine head and neck tissue to simulate a variety of procedures including blepharoplasty, ptosis repair, orbital floor exploration, facial nerve dissection and repair, mandibular plating, tracheotomy, laryngofissure, tracheal resection, and laryngectomy. The authors found this simulator to be anatomically compatible, affordable, and useful for a variety of procedures.

There are several additional head and neck surgery physical simulators. Simulators for microvascular anastomosis have involved animal models, such as chicken thigh vasculature. However, there are also commercially available synthetic materials that simulate vasculature and have been used in our bootcamps to teach vascular repair, such as internal jugular vein repair. By including IV tubing and red-dyed fluid, active bleeding is also simulated. Additionally, we have used commercially available simulated bowel sections for teaching the inverting Connell stitch, commonly used in total laryngectomies. Impressively, Griffin and colleagues[53] reported the first published neck dissection simulator in which they use a blue phantom central line placement training model and modify it such that a selective neck dissection could be performed using real surgical instruments, complete with vascular and neural structures commonly encountered during a neck dissection. A robotic surgical simulator proposed by Sperry and colleagues[54] involves the da Vinci Robot (Intuitive Surgical Inc, Sunnyvale, CA) and a cadaveric head to complete dissections for preparation of performing a radical tonsillectomy, supraglottic partial laryngectomy, and base of tongue resection.

Rigid esophagoscopy is an important skill for residents to master. Recently, a group engineered a rigid esophagoscopy model with force sensors under the maxillary incisor and at the tip of the esophagoscope.[55]

VIRTUAL-REALITY SIMULATORS

In contrast to physical simulators, virtual-reality simulators in otolaryngology provide computer-generated environments that have anatomic visual representations. These virtual-reality simulators can include two-dimensional or more commonly 3D representations of a surgical environment or setting. Advancement in engineering and computer technologies has allowed for the incorporation of sensory feedback that can enhance the simulator's capacity to mimic real-life situations and experiences. For example, with temporal bone simulators, besides the 3D visual interfaces, haptic feedback provides tactile feel and auditory input (the sound of drilling) and can make the experience more lifelike and immersive.

Virtual-reality simulators require expert teams of engineers, computer scientists, and medical professionals to create these sophisticated systems. This engineering investment and the requirement to purchase technology can make these virtual-reality systems costly. Otolaryngology is a small medical specialty, thus large-scale production of a virtual-reality simulator for a specialized application may not be profitable for investors. This is a significant barrier to development and dissemination of this technology.

Airway and Laryngeal Virtual-Reality Simulators

The sole airway virtual-reality simulator available involves virtual bronchoscopic models that simulate flexible bronchoscopy with accurate distal airway anatomy (See **Table 1**).[1,56–60] Some systems are capable of haptic feedback. Additionally, some of these virtual-reality simulators are available for purchase. The commercialization of this virtual-reality simulator is likely caused by its broader application beyond just otolaryngology to pulmonary and perhaps anesthesia. Furthermore, there is a Web site that provides the learner with an opportunity to explore virtual bronchoscopy using real-time video for free.[61] The learner engages in short video segments through the computer's mouse/trackpad. Although the procedural realism is limited, this still has a role for the novice to learn the bronchial anatomy.

Otology Physical Virtual-Reality Simulators

Otology as a subspecialty has some of the most well designed and validated virtual-reality simulators (See **Table 2**). One of the most important skills for medical students and otolaryngology residents to master is otoscopy. It is critical to properly identify normal versus pathologic findings on examinations. OtoSim (OtoSim Inc, Toronto, Canada) is a commercially available otoscopy simulator that uses a physical/realistic model ear and otoscope with high-fidelity images of tympanic membranes and middle ear pathology. Another version simulates pneumatic otoscopy. In a study using the OtoSim, 93% of medical students reported increased confidence in otoscopy skills after using OtoSim.[62]

Virtual-reality simulators exist for myringotomy,[63] with some also incorporating haptic feedback.[64,65] As virtual-reality simulators, these systems require specialized computer programming and hardware. Concerns of poor haptic feedback and face validity exist.

Temporal bone drilling is perhaps the area in otology with the most development in terms of virtual-reality simulation. There are a myriad of validated virtual-reality temporal bone simulators including the VOXEL-MAN, Mediseus temporal bone simulator, Ohio State University Simulator, and Stanford Temporal Bone surgical.[66–69] Technological advancements have led to incremental improvements in the virtual-reality technology used in these systems. These systems use the PHANTOM haptic device for feedback and 3D visual interfaces to allow a more realistic feel. The VOXEL-MAN, Ohio State University Simulator, and the Mediseus temporal bone simulators are probably the three most well studied. From personal experience, the Ohio State University Simulator allows an immersive experience with audiologic drill sounds, haptic feedback, varied pathologies, and even training modules that evaluate and provide feedback for the trainee. A recent review of virtual-reality in otolaryngology concluded that a temporal bone virtual-reality platform is worthy of incorporating into training programs especially in the early years, but that real-life operative experience cannot be replaced.[70] These systems allow unlimited repetition, improved understanding of surgical anatomy, and can facilitate surgical planning.

Sinus/Rhinology Virtual-Reality Simulators

Sinus procedures lend themselves to virtual-reality simulation because sinus tissues, like temporal bone tissues, are less vulnerable to deformation and thus less burdensome to model from a computational point of view.[71] In addition, sinus procedures rely heavily on instrumentation, thus enabling ease of motion-tracking for performance analysis and feedback (See **Table 3**).

Among the earliest and well-described virtual-reality simulators is the nasal endoscopy simulator.[72] A head model coupled with a graphics workstation uses image data sets of the nasal cavity and paranasal sinus area from previous patients. A tracking system measures the position of the endoscope and surgical instruments in space, and provides formative feedback for basic procedures.[72] Initially, a limitation was the lack of proprioceptive feedback, hence subsequent models have incorporated haptics.[73,74]

Soon thereafter, the Endoscopic Sinus Surgery Simulator (ES3), developed by Lockheed Martin (Lockheed Martin, Bethesda, MD),[71] demonstrated enhanced capabilities. The hardware included four components: a workstation simulation platform (Silicon Graphics Inc, Mountain View, CA); a personal computer–based haptic controller; a personal computer–based voice-recognition-enabled instructor that operated the simulator through spoken commands; and an electromechanical human interaction platform with replica of an endoscope, surgical tool handle, and rubber-headed mannequin. This simulator provided training for scope manipulation, mucosal injection, middle turbinate medialization, uncinectomy, and maxillary antrostomy, all requiring ambidexterity, navigation in 3D space, and technical accuracy. A rigorous modified Delphi method with participation from experts in otolaryngology, surgical education, statistical analysis, behavioral science, and simulator development was used to define performance metrics.[75] A list of error categories was generated and discussed individually until consensus was reached on each error attribute, classification, measurement, and reporting standard. The simulator collected and analyzed performance data using these standards throughout trainee use, and could provide formative feedback in real time. It also archived the data to provide summative information for performance evaluation and reporting.[75,76]

Beyond a meticulous design, the ES3 is among the most extensively validated sinus simulators. ES3 trainee performance has been shown to correlate strongly with visuospatial perception as measured by scores on the previously validated Pictorial Surface Orientation simulator,[77] which requires trainees to orient an arrow perpendicular to a cube using cursor keys and has been shown to predict laparoscopic performance.[78] Concurrent, discriminant, and construct validity have been demonstrated through multi-institutional studies involving subjects ranging from novices to experts.[76,79] Predictive validity has been shown with improved overall procedure time, reduced errors, and greater instrument manipulation dexterity on various endoscopic tasks.[80] Finally, trainees have been shown to demonstrate skill retention over the moderate term (average, 35 days) compared with control subjects.[81] Despite this painstaking design, development, and validation, as with other virtual-reality sinus simulators, commercial development for the ES3 has been curtailed by a small market and high development costs.

Miscellaneous Virtual-Reality Simulators

With the widespread dissemination of robotic surgery into otolaryngology, it is essential that residents gain appropriate training in this novel modality (See **Table 4**). The da Vinci Skills Simulator (Intuitive Surgical Inc) teaches residents basic maneuvering and operation of the robot.[82–84] Instead of surgical procedures, this simulator uses the da Vinci controls and interface to navigate in a virtual-reality world to complete tasks, such as camera targeting, placing objects on a matchboard, ring and rail, needle targeting, and energy dissection.

With the increasing number of subtotal/intracapsular tonsillectomies being performed, there has even been a virtual-reality simulator with haptic feedback reported for this procedure.[85] Visual and auditory cues were used to alert the user when critical structures, such as the tonsil capsule, were approached or breached. The haptic device mimicked a Coblation handpiece. Further validation studies are needed with this prototype.

A virtual-reality simulator for fine-needle aspiration biopsy has been reported for lesions in the thyroid.[86]

REFERENCES

1. Deutsch ES, Christenson T, Curry J, et al. Multimodality education for airway endoscopy skill development. Ann Otol Rhinol Laryngol 2009;118:81–6.
2. Ianacone DC, Gnadt BJ, Isaacson G. Ex vivo ovine model for head and neck surgical simulation. Am J Otolaryngol 2016;37:272–8.
3. Howells TH, Emery FM, Twentyman JE. Endotracheal intubation training using a simulator: an evaluation of the Laerdal adult intubation model in the teaching of endotracheal intubation. Br J Anaesth 1973;45:400–2.
4. Hesselfeldt R, Kristensen MS, Rasmussen LS. Evaluation of the airway of the SimMan full-scale patient simulator. Acta Anaesthesiol Scand 2005;49: 1339–45.
5. Schebesta K, Hupfl M, Ringl H, et al. A comparison of paediatric airway anatomy with the SimBaby high-fidelity patient simulator. Resuscitation 2011;82: 468–72.

6. Sawyer T, Strandjord TP, Johnson K, et al. Neonatal airway simulators, how good are they? A comparative study of physical and functional fidelity. J Perinatol 2016; 36:151–6.

7. Latif R, Bautista A, Duan X, et al. Teaching advanced airway management skills: using simulation to accelerate the fiberoptic intubation learning curve. Crit Care Med 2010;38:A134.

8. Smith ME, Leung BC, Sharma R, et al. A randomized controlled trial of nasolaryngoscopy training techniques. Laryngoscope 2014;124:2034–8.

9. Amin M, Rosen CA, Simpson CB, et al. Hands-on training methods for vocal fold injection education. Ann Otol Rhinol Laryngol 2007;116:1–6.

10. Dedmon MM, Paddle PM, Phillips J, et al. Development and validation of a high-fidelity porcine laryngeal surgical simulator. Otolaryngol Head Neck Surg 2015; 153:420–6.

11. Awad Z, Patel B, Hayden L, et al. Simulation in laryngology training; what should we invest in? Our experience with 64 porcine larynges and a literature review. Clin Otolaryngol 2015;40:269–73.

12. Nixon IJ, Palmer FL, Ganly I, et al. An integrated simulator for endolaryngeal surgery. Laryngoscope 2012;122:140–3.

13. Fleming J, Kapoor K, Sevdalis N, et al. Validation of an operating room immersive microlaryngoscopy simulator. Laryngoscope 2012;122:1099–103.

14. Contag SP, Klein AM, Blount AC, et al. Validation of a laryngeal dissection module for phonomicrosurgical training. Laryngoscope 2009;119:211–5.

15. Holliday MA, Bones VM, Malekzadeh S, et al. Low-cost modular phonosurgery training station: development and validation. Laryngoscope 2015;125:1409–13.

16. Cabrera-Muffly C, Clary MS, Abaza M. A low-cost transcervical laryngeal injection trainer. Laryngoscope 2016;126:901–5.

17. Ainsworth TA, Kobler JB, Loan GJ, et al. Simulation model for transcervical laryngeal injection providing real-time feedback. Ann Otol Rhinol Laryngol 2014;123: 881–6.

18. Ross PD, Steven R, Zhang D, et al. Computer-assessed performance of psychomotor skills in endoscopic otolaryngology surgery: construct validity of the Dundee Endoscopic Psychomotor Otolaryngology Surgery Trainer (DEPOST). Surg Endosc 2015;29:3125–31.

19. Volsky PG, Hughley BB, Peirce SM, et al. Construct validity of a simulator for myringotomy with ventilation tube insertion. Otolaryngol Head Neck Surg 2009;141: 603–8.

20. Malekzadeh S, Hanna G, Wilson B, et al. A model for training and evaluation of myringotomy and tube placement skills. Laryngoscope 2011;121:1410–5.

21. Hong P, Webb AN, Corsten G, et al. An anatomically sound surgical simulation model for myringotomy and tympanostomy tube insertion. Int J Pediatr Otorhinolaryngol 2014;78:522–9.

22. Estomba C, García JMM, Zavarce MIH, et al. The Vigo grommet trainer. Eur Ann Otorhinolaryngol Head Neck Dis 2015;132:53–5.

23. Mills R, Lee P. Surgical skills training in middle-ear surgery. J Laryngol Otol 2003; 117:159–63.

24. Monfared A, Mitteramskogler G, Grube S, et al. High-fidelity, inexpensive surgical middle ear simulator. Otol Neurotol 2012;33:1573–7.

25. Clark MPA, Westerberg BD, Mitchell JE. Development and validation of a low cost microsurgery ear trainer for low-resource settings. J Laryngol Otol 2016;130: 954–61.

26. Barber SR, Kozin ED, Dedmon M, et al. 3D-printed pediatric endoscopic ear surgery simulator for surgical training. Int J Pediatr Otorhinolaryngol 2016;90:113–8.
27. Anschuetz L, Bonali M, Ghirelli M, et al. An ovine model for exclusive endoscopic ear surgery. JAMA Otolaryngol Head Neck Surg 2016;143(3):247–52.
28. Awad Z, Ahmed S, Taghi AS, et al. Feasibility of a synthetic temporal bone for training in mastoidectomy: face, content, and concurrent validity. Otol Neurotol 2014;35:1813–8.
29. Da Cruz MJ, Francis HW. Face and content validation of a novel three-dimensional printed temporal bone for surgical skills development. J Laryngol Otol 2015;129(Suppl 3):S23–9.
30. Mick PT, Arnoldner C, Mainprize JG, et al. Face validity study of an artificial temporal bone for simulation surgery. Otol Neurotol 2013;34:1305–10.
31. Mowry SE, Jammal H, Myer C, et al. A novel temporal bone simulation model using 3d printing techniques. Otol Neurotol 2015;36:1562–5.
32. Hochman JB, Rhodes C, Wong D, et al. Comparison of cadaveric and isomorphic three-dimensional printed models in temporal bone education. Laryngoscope 2015;125:2353–7.
33. Rose AS, Kimbell JS, Webster CE, et al. Multi-material 3d models for temporal bone surgical simulation. Ann Otol Rhinol Laryngol 2015;124:528–36.
34. Tolisano AM, Justin GA, Ruhl DS, et al. Rhinology and medical malpractice: an update of the medicolegal landscape of the last ten years. Laryngoscope 2016;126:14–9.
35. Awad Z, Touska P, Arora A, et al. Face and content validity of sheep heads in endoscopic rhinology training. Int Forum Allergy Rhinol 2014;4:851–8.
36. Malekzadeh S, Pfisterer MJ, Wilson B, et al. A novel low-cost sinus surgery task trainer. Otolaryngol Head Neck Surg 2011;145:530–3.
37. Steehler MK, Chu EE, Na H, et al. Teaching and assessing endoscopic sinus surgery skills on a validated low-cost task trainer. Laryngoscope 2013;123:841–4.
38. Harbison RA, Johnson KE, Miller C, et al. Face, content, and construct validation of a low-cost, non-biologic, sinus surgery task trainer and knowledge-based curriculum. Int Forum Allergy Rhinol 2017;7(4):405–13.
39. Scott GM, Roth K, Rotenberg B, et al. Evaluation of a novel high-fidelity epistaxis task trainer. Laryngoscope 2016;126:1501–3.
40. Pettineo CM, Vozenilek JA, Kharasch M, et al. Epistaxis simulator: an innovative design. Simul Healthc 2008;3:239–41.
41. Malekzadeh S, Deutsch ES, Malloy KM. Simulation-based otorhinolaryngology emergencies boot camp: Part 2: special skills using task trainers. Laryngoscope 2014;124:1566–9.
42. Pearson CR, Wallace HC. The tonsil cup: a simple teaching aid for tonsillectomy. J Laryngol Otol 1997;111:1064–5.
43. Duodu J, Lesser THJ. Tonsil tie simulator. J Laryngol Otol 2013;127:924–6.
44. Raja MK, Haneefa MA, Chidambaram A. Yorick's skull model for tonsillectomy tie training. Clin Otolaryngol 2008;33:187–8.
45. Street I, Beech T, Jennings C. The Birmingham trainer: a simulator for ligating the lower tonsillar pole. Clin Otolaryngol 2006;31:79.
46. Bunting H, Wilson BM, Malloy KM, et al. A novel peritonsillar abscess simulator. Simul Healthc 2015;10:320–5.
47. Scott GM, Fung K, Roth KE. Novel high-fidelity peritonsillar abscess simulator. Otolaryngol Head Neck Surg 2016;154:634–7.
48. Taylor SR, Chang CWD. Novel peritonsillar abscess task simulator. Otolaryngol Head Neck Surg 2014;151:10–3.

49. Giblett N, Hari C. Introducing a realistic and reusable quinsy simulator. J Laryngol Otol 2016;30:201–3.
50. Janus JR, Hamilton GS. The use of open-cell foam and elastic foam tape as an affordable skin simulator for teaching suture technique. JAMA Facial Plast Surg 2013;15:385–7.
51. Gilmour A, Taghizadeh R, Payne CE. The educational hand and head: novel teaching tools in the design and execution of local flaps. J Plast Reconstr Aesthet Surg 2012;65:981–2.
52. Taylor SR, Chang DCW. Gelatin facial skin simulator for cutaneous reconstruction. Otolaryngol Head Neck Surg 2016;154:279–81.
53. Griffin GR, Rosenbaum S, Hecht S, et al. Development of a moderate fidelity neck dissection simulator. Laryngoscope 2013;123:1682–5.
54. Sperry SM, O'Malley BW Jr, Weinstein GS. The University of Pennsylvania curriculum for training otorhinolaryngology residents in transoral robotic surgery. ORL J Otorhinolaryngol Relat Spec 2014;76:342–52.
55. Allak A, Liu YE, Oliynyk MS, et al. Development and evaluation of a rigid esophagoscopy simulator for residency training. Laryngoscope 2016;126:616–9.
56. Mandal S, Patel ARC, Goldring JJP. A simulated bronchoscopy course for new specialist trainees. Thorax 2010;65:A117.
57. Patel ARC, Mandal S, Goldring JJP. Simulated bronchoscopy training delivered by experienced peers improves confidence of new trainees. Thorax 2010;65:A116.
58. Pastis NJ, Vanderbilt AA, Tanner NT, et al. Construct validity of the Simbionix Bronch mentor simulator for essential bronchoscopic skills. J Bronchology Interv Pulmonol 2014;21:314–21.
59. Vaidyanath C, Sharma M, Mistry V, et al. ORSIM™ bronchoscopy simulator improves psychomotor skills for fibreoptic intubation amongst novices. Br J Anaesth 2013;111:691P.
60. Rowe R, Cohen RA. An evaluation of a virtual reality airway simulator. Anesth Analg 2002;95:62–6.
61. Available at: http://www.thoracic-anesthesia.com/. Accessed December 20, 2016.
62. Lee DJ, Fu TS, Carrillo B, et al. Evaluation of an otoscopy simulator to teach otoscopy and normative anatomy to first year medical students. Laryngoscope 2015;125:2159–62.
63. Wheeler B, Doyle PC, Chandarana S, et al. Interactive computer-based simulator for training in blade navigation and targeting in myringotomy. Comput Methods Programs Biomed 2010;98:130–9.
64. Sowerby LJ, Rehal G, Husein M, et al. Development and face validity testing of a three-dimensional myringotomy simulator with haptic feedback. J Otolaryngol Head Neck Surg 2010;39:122–9.
65. Ho AK, Alsaffar H, Doyle PC, et al. Virtual reality myringotomy simulation with real-time deformation: development and validity testing. Laryngoscope 2012;122:1844–51.
66. Zirkle M, Roberson DW, Leuwer R, et al. Using a virtual reality temporal bone simulator to assess otolaryngology trainees. Laryngoscope 2007;117:258–63.
67. Wiet GJ, Stredney D, Sessanna D, et al. Virtual temporal bone dissection: an interactive surgical simulator. Otolaryngol Head Neck Surg 2002;127:79–83.
68. Sewell C, Morris D, Blevins NH, et al. Providing metrics and performance feedback in a surgical simulator. Comput Aided Surg 2008;13:63–81.

69. Zhao YC, Kennedy G, Yukawa K, et al. Can virtual reality simulator be used as a training aid to improve cadaver temporal bone dissection? results of a randomized blinded control trial. Laryngoscope 2011;121:831–7.
70. Arora A, Lau LYM, Awad Z, et al. Virtual reality simulation training in otolaryngology. Int J Surg 2014;12:87–94.
71. Edmond CV Jr. Impact of the endoscopic sinus surgical simulator on operating room performance. Laryngoscope 2002;112:1148–58.
72. Ecke U, Klimek L, Müller W, et al. Virtual reality: preparation and execution of sinus surgery. Comput Aided Surg 1998;3:45–50.
73. Caversaccio M, Eichenberger A, Häusler R. Virtual simulator as a training tool for endonasal surgery. Am J Rhinol 2003;17:283–90.
74. Tolsdorff B, Pommert A, Höhne KH, et al. Virtual reality: a new paranasal sinus surgery simulator. Laryngoscope 2010;120:420–6.
75. Satava RM, Fried MP. A methodology for objective assessment of errors: an example using an endoscopic sinus surgery simulator. Otolaryngol Clin North Am 2002;35:1289–301.
76. Fried MP, Sadoughi B, Weghorst SJ, et al. Construct validity of the endoscopic sinus surgery simulator: II. Assessment of discriminant validity and expert benchmarking. Arch Otolaryngol Head Neck Surg 2007;133:350–7.
77. Arora H, Uribe J, Ralph W, et al. Assessment of construct validity of the endoscopic sinus surgery simulator. Arch Otolaryngol Head Neck Surg 2005;131:217–21.
78. Gallagher AG, Cowie R, Crothers I, et al. PicSOr: an objective test of perceptual skill that predicts laparoscopic technical skill in three initial studies of laparoscopic performance. Surg Endosc 2003;17:1468–71.
79. Fried MP, Satava R, Weghorst S, et al. Identifying and reducing errors with surgical simulation. Qual Saf Health Care 2004;13(Suppl 1):19–26.
80. Fried MP, Sadoughi B, Gibber MJ, et al. From virtual reality to the operating room: the endoscopic sinus surgery simulator experiment. Otolaryngol Head Neck Surg 2010;142:202–7.
81. Uribe JI, Ralph WM Jr, Glaser AY, et al. Learning curves, acquisition, and retention of skills trained with the endoscopic sinus surgery simulator. Am J Rhinol 2004;18:87–92.
82. Walliczek U, Förtsch A, Dworschak P, et al. Effect of training frequency on the learning curve on the da Vinci Skills Simulator. Head and Neck 2016;38(Suppl 1):E1762–9.
83. Walliczek-Dworschak U, Mandapathil M, Förtsch A, et al. Structured training on the da Vinci Skills Simulator leads to improvement in technical performance of robotic novices. Clin Otolaryngol 2017;42:71–80.
84. Zhang N, Sumer BD. Transoral robotic surgery: simulation-based standardized training. JAMA Otolaryngol Head Neck Surg 2013;139:1111–7.
85. Ruthenbeck GS, Tan SB, Carney AS, et al. A virtual-reality subtotal tonsillectomy simulator. J Laryngol Otol 2012;126(Suppl S2):S8–13.
86. Souza IA, Sanches C, Zuffo MK. Virtual reality simulator for training of needle biopsy of thyroid gland nodules. Med Meets Virtual Reality 2009;17:352–7.

Improving Rhinology Skills with Simulation

Andrew Y. Lee, MD, Marvin P. Fried, MD, Marc Gibber, MD*

KEYWORDS

- Endoscopic sinus surgery simulation • Rhinology simulation • Simulation training
- Virtual reality • Surgical rehearsal • Medical technology

KEY POINTS

- The use of surgical simulators in teaching residents the basic technical foundation and skills necessary to be proficient in rhinological surgery before operating on the live patient is discussed.
- An overview is given of both high-fidelity and low-fidelity rhinological simulators, and the keys to development of novel and validated simulators are highlighted.
- The importance of the combination of high-fidelity and low-fidelity simulators on maximizing resident education and training in rhinological surgery is clarified.

INTRODUCTION

With the advent of work-restriction hours and limited time availability for training surgical residents in light of increased scrutiny in providing excellent patient care with reduced risk, it's become increasingly important to find novel and efficient ways of improving the surgical knowledge and skill of residents. Surgical simulation allows trainees the opportunity to hone their skills in a standardized and monitored environment before applying the skills on a patient. Simulation has many benefits including (Brandon Hall Research News, 2005)

- It provides a safe environment for the trainee to make mistakes
- It significantly reduces training time by creating the most efficient path to solving specific problems
- The student may practice procedures such as flying in hazardous conditions
- Creation of simulations leads to improvements in the process and can help streamline the processes being taught
- There is significant retention of the simulation procedures

Disclosure Statement: No disclosures to report.
Department of Otorhinolaryngology–Head and Neck Surgery, Montefiore Medical Center, Albert Einstein College of Medicine, 3400 Bainbridge Avenue, 3rd Floor, Bronx, NY 14067, USA
* Corresponding author.
E-mail address: mgibber@montefiore.org

Otolaryngol Clin N Am 50 (2017) 893–901
http://dx.doi.org/10.1016/j.otc.2017.05.002
0030-6665/17/© 2017 Elsevier Inc. All rights reserved.

- The modeling of expert behaviors during simulation training helps transfer expert thinking to the trainee
- Cost efficiency of simulations allows the user the ability to practice without risk of damaging or pulling expensive equipment offline.

Medical-simulation validation studies have shown that the skills learned by trainees using a simulator have significant improved student's performances by decreasing operating times, decreasing errors, and improving efficiency, ultimately reducing the time to proficiency and improving overall patient safety.[1] High-fidelity medical simulations that allow surgeons to perform procedures before doing the same procedure on a patient have shown to have great impact on skills training and learning.[2] The resident is allowed to make mistakes and learn from them in a simulated environment without compromising patient safety.

Surgical rhinology, which is predominately performed endoscopically, lends itself to a variety of innovative and creative ways to teach residents outside of the operating room. One such way is through virtual reality, which has been shown to be an important tool for medical and surgical training and education in a variety of fields.[3–7] It has provided residents an introduction to a wide breadth of laparoscopic, gastrointestinal, plastic, ophthalmologic, dermatologic, urologic, and laryngological procedures.[8–15]

Rhinological simulation not only allows students to practice and learn the procedure and anatomy[15,16] but can also help train and reinforce trainees comfort level with, technique, and various rhinological instruments and their correct application. Overall, this increases the resident's proficiency in performing simple to complex rhinological procedures before patient care.[17]

HISTORY OF SIMULATION IN RHINOLOGY

The practice of simulation has been around for centuries, particularly in the military field in which simulation has been used to practice skills, problem solving, and judgment.[18] It was not until the twentieth century that human patient simulation helped to evolve medical learning and practice,[18] and increased the intensity of medical training through simulation, similar to other fields such as aviation and the military.[19]

Given the advent of endoscopic techniques and its effectiveness in nasal and paranasal sinus surgery, the need for training surgeons capable of operating with the endoscope and surgical tools in a complex anatomic environment was of utmost importance.[20] From 1995 to 1998, collaboration between multiple institutions and The Lockheed Martin Corporation produced the first virtual reality simulator in endoscopic sinus surgery, the endoscopic sinus surgery simulator (ES3).[21] The ES3 established simulation training in endoscopic sinus surgery and set the trend for the development of future rhinological simulators.

VALIDATION

The validation of surgical simulators plays a vital role in their acceptance as effective training tools. Though the process of validation has been extensively discussed elsewhere,[22] numerous validation benchmarks are currently used with the most subjective validation benchmarks being used in the initial phases of test construction. The various validation benchmarks include

- Face validity and content validity: rely on input of experts to determine whether the contents of the test are appropriate and cohesive
- Concurrent validity: compare existing training curriculums or current gold standard assessments to those of the simulator

- Discriminant validity: focus on whether the scores generated by the simulator correlate accurately with appropriate factors and can stratify subjects into appropriate score levels
- Predictive validity: typically, the final benchmark test that determines whether scores on the simulator accurately predict real skill performance.

SIMULATORS IN ENDOSCOPIC SINUS SURGERY

The challenge facing trainees in becoming proficient in endoscopic sinus surgery is overwhelming and extends beyond the complexities of the actual procedure itself. The beginner trainee must also learn

- The intricate 3-dimensional (D) anatomy of the nasal cavity and paranasal sinuses
- Translating 2D visualization into the anatomic 3D space
- Spatial awareness and bimanual dexterity in working with the endoscope and surgical instruments
- Proper body positioning of not only themselves but also the patient
- Decision-making process for selecting proper surgical instrumentation to complete the intended task.

Simulators have allowed the student the ability to practice these skills repeatedly without compromising patient care and safety.[23] Furthermore, the student and the teacher can objectively assess surgical skills and progression in a quantifiable manner by looking at surgical metrics and correcting deficiencies.[24] As new state of the art simulators continue to be developed, they can be used to teach basic skills through repetitive procedures, allowing for the detection and analysis of surgical errors and near-miss incidents without risk to the patient.[25,26] **Box 1** is a consensus list of errors identified in endoscopic sinus surgery that can be used to examine and track student progression.[24]

Software Development

One of the difficulties in creating surgical simulators is making the simulator multisensory while including realistic visualizations and haptic interactions. The goal is to provide the physician with patient-specific realizations of anatomy and physiology while being fluid enough to modify the visual appearance as the student interacts with the environment (eg, through injections, incisions, bleeding, resections, ablations, deformations). Furthermore, the haptic feedback should give the student the feel of the instruments as they interact with the rigid and nonrigid structures within the environment.[24]

Specific to rhinology and endoscopic sinus surgery, the development of realistic simulators is vital in preparing students to operate effectively when faced with the actual patient. Given the complexity of the anatomic structures confined within such a small space, there is a steep learning curve for trainees learning to develop bimanual skills with control of the endoscope and instrument. Effective simulators can be developed to focus on individual components of the procedure (ie, introduction of instruments through the nasal vestibule, driving the endoscope, or instrumentation of the maxillary ostium) or attempt to encompass the entirety of the procedure.

Diagnostic images of patients can be used to derive visual and haptic realization of a simulator, particularly as they relate to the nasal cavity and paranasal sinuses. Computed tomography (CT) imagery of the sinuses can effectively separate the large cortical bone from the surrounding soft tissue and air passages. Given that the

Box 1
Taxonomy of errors in endoscopic sinus surgery

Technical

Scope handling
- Scope dirty
- Tool: scope collision
- Contact with the wall
- Repetitive scope insertion
- Bleeding obscuring view
- Improper insertion of scope
- Wandering scope unstable

Instrument handling
- Mucosal injury (tissue report)
- Dissection error
- Past pointing
- Instrument out of view

Controlling field of view
- Lack of perspective
- Image task alignment

Cognitive

Know anatomy
- Misidentifying (anatomic recognition)
- Incomplete examination (leaving out steps)

Know instruments
- Wrong tool choice
- Wrong scope choice

Know procedure sequences
- Task out of sequence
- Omit a step
- Lack of progress

Know procedure technique
- Improper exposure
- Wandering scope: not recognizing a target

Not recognizing an injury
- Artery injury
- Bleeding

Combined

Over or under dissection (improper tissue resection)
  Injuries
  - Orbital injury
  - Cranial nerve injury
  - Lamina papyracea
  - Cribriform plate injury
  - Lacrimal system injury
  - Destabilization of the middle turbinate

Improper location of injection

Rotation (navigation)

From Satava RM, Fried MP. A methodology for objective assessment of errors: an example using an endoscopic sinus surgery simulator. Otolaryngol Clin North Am 2002;35(6):1296; with permission.

standard before undergoing sinus surgery is obtaining a CT scan of the sinuses, individualized patient-specific models can be generated for the simulator, allowing surgeons to rehearse the procedure specific to the patient's anatomy.[24]

Visualization Software Development

The mucosa of the nasal cavity and paranasal sinuses are prone to bleeding with frequent need of suctioning and placement of vasoconstrictive agents to gain adequate visualization during the procedure. The simulation of realistic bleeding is difficult, but efforts focused on visually emulating the complex anatomy and tissue interactions would provide students with an advanced realism in their training.

The Human Interface Technology Laboratory, at the University of Washington, has developed a video-texture approach[14] to portray bleeding. This technique was developed to support the representation of blood flow during a simulated transurethral resection of the prostate procedure, in which control of excessive bleeding is a concern. Videos were acquired in vitro from an endoscopic view of a physical tube into which red fluid was injected at varying rates and angles. The alpha-mapped video segments were then looped to create a seamless pulsating bleeder, which could then be placed (algorithmically or manually) into the virtual prostate anatomy. Trainees were able to handle bleeders either by increasing the fluid flow through the resectoscope or by electrocautery. Similarly, sources of bleeding can be diffuse, which will require broad hemostatic or focal (ie, specific vessel) procedures, which would be an entirely different surgical approach. Other models used to produce realistic bleeding focus on the use of particle-based methods that exploit the vertex shaders available on the current-generation graphics card.[23]

The Endoscopic Sinus Surgery Simulator

The ES3 was among the first sinus surgery virtual reality simulators and has been studied and validated to affect resident training.[27] Based on aviation models, the ES3 simulator was developed using both visual and haptic (force) feedback in a virtual reality environment.[15,28,29] It was designed as a procedural simulator that trains and assesses the performance of an entire task that requires navigation, ambidexterity, and accuracy, and allows for analysis of these tasks. The simulator has 4 main components:

- SGI Octane workstation (Silicon Graphics Inc, Mountain View, CA, USA) that serves as the simulation host platform
- Computer-based haptic controlling that provides control and coordination between a universal physical instrument handle and a set of virtual surgical instruments
- Computer-based voice recognition-enabled instructor that operates the simulator by responding to spoken commands
- An electromechanical platform that serves as the human interaction interface with an endoscope, surgical tool handle, and rubber-headed mannequin.[30]

The ES3 has been assessed for both construct and predictive validity. In a study looking at construct validity, the performance of students on the ES3 simulator correlated strongly with their scores on previously validated measures of perceptual, visuospatial, and psychomotor performance.[20] Furthermore, in a follow-up study focusing on discriminant validity, the simulator was shown to train novice subjects to attain expert surgeon benchmark performance criteria and performances near that of experience sinus surgeons, with retention of those skills.[30,31] The ES3 has also shown to be effective in translating the skills learned on the simulator to actual patient care,[27,32] which is the primary goal of simulator training.

Although the use and availability of the ES3 simulator is restricted, the impact of the simulator in sinus surgery training cannot be overstated and provides a framework and foundation of evidence supporting the use of surgical simulators in endoscopic sinus training. Residents may range in inherent skills or abilities, with students starting at different levels, but the outcome for each individual training on the simulator translates to at least equal, if not superior, operative performance compared with the finite repetition of live surgical procedures.[32]

Other Sinus Surgery Simulators

With the limited use and high cost of the ES3 simulator, the development of newer simulators that can affect resident training have been researched and developed. Simulators such as the Dextroscope endoscopic sinus simulator (Dextroscope endoscopic sinus simulator, Volume interactions),[3] VOXEL-MAN simulator,[33] and McGill Simulator for Endoscopic Sinus Surgery[34] are some of the virtual reality simulators available for endoscopic sinus surgery training. The McGill simulator for endoscopic sinus surgery aims to combine novel tools with elaborate anatomic deformities in a realistic platform and has shown promising initial results in resident training.[34,35] These new high-fidelity simulators have improved haptic feedback and created more of a life-like environment with improvements in high-definition visualization, as well as prevented students from penetrating through anatomic structures. A novel aspect of the McGill simulator is the addition of blurring of the monitor when the endoscopic tip becomes soiled, forcing the user to be more aware of the endoscope in relation to the surrounding anatomy.[35] Furthermore, as technology continues to improve, these simulators allow for tissue deformity and dynamic movement of the structures, giving a more realistic feel to the surgical environment.

Though the focus has been primarily on virtual reality simulators, another simulator type involves real anatomic models. One such simulator is the Sinus Model Otorhino Neuro Trainer (Sinus Model Otorhino Neuro Trainer, nogueira et al), which was based of images of anatomic structures, CT, and endoscopic anatomic dissection videos of cadavers to create a real anatomic model.[36]

Low-Fidelity Simulators

Low-fidelity simulators can play an important role in endoscopic training, particularly in the beginner rhinologist. A large hurdle in the ability to integrate simulator training into resident training is the extensive cost of more high-fidelity sinus surgery simulators. Simulators using low-cost, basic tools can help teach these basic skills before advancing to more complex procedures. One such inexpensive simulator developed at Georgetown University constructed a training model using gelatin and reusable, recyclable, and readily available materials for less than 5 US dollars that resulted in improved camera skills, instrumentation, and hand-eye coordination.[37]

The authors' institution has implemented a low-fidelity rhinological simulator in conjunction with the Department of Orthopedics to expose junior residents to the basics of endoscopic surgery using various vegetables as mediums to simulate the nasal cavity. This teaches the student proper handling of the endoscope and allows them the ability to practice dexterity with the camera and to learn to be spatially aware while working in a 3D space when looking on a 2D screen. Another study that looked at the use of low-fidelity training models using low-cost, easily constructed modules and its impact on 5 novice and 9 senior residents found a statistically more significant improvement in performance in the module-training group than in the nontraining group.[38]

Although lacking the ability to teach or practice more complex and advanced procedures, the overall impact of the use of low-fidelity simulators in rhinological training cannot be underestimated, particularly focusing on the development of a basic surgical foundation.

SUMMARY

Surgical simulators in the training of otorhinolaryngology residents continues to evolve and can play a vital role in preparing residents before treating patients. As more realistic simulators are developed and implemented into resident curriculums, students will be able to develop procedural skills in an objectively assessed and educational environment. Skill acquisition and development through the simulator will provide students with the basic foundations and allow them to repeatedly focus on certain aspects of their abilities that may be lacking without compromising patient care, particularly in the rhinological field in which almost all procedures are done using endoscopic techniques. In the age of work hour restrictions, simulation training enables the trainee to increase the number of cases they do, whether in basic sinus surgery or more advanced skull base surgery. This allows them to obtain extensive operating room time before any live surgical activity.

To acquire these skills, low fidelity, cost-effective simulators allow students to acquire basic technical skills from learning instruments to driving the camera. As the student progresses, the addition of high-fidelity simulators allows the learner to apply the basic technical skills they practice to more realistic scenarios and cases. As both the high-fidelity and low-fidelity models become more sophisticated, students will be able to further improve their basic skills with further realistic repetitions of surgical cases that will make them more comfortable doing the procedure, and give the mentor more reassurance in the resident's skills.

The ultimate use of these devices will be to download the actual patient sinus CT into a simulator and then to perform a mission rehearsal on the patient's actual anatomy and pathologic condition before taking the patient to the operating room. Moreover, critical areas, such as the cranial base and orbit, can be annotated at the rehearsal and can be used intraoperatively to warn of these close relationships during surgery. The extent of the pathologic condition can also be assessed before the procedure. In addition, the scans can be developed into a teaching library to be used by multiple trainees.

The use of simulators in rhinology will continue to allow the rapid development of skills from the junior to the more senior level in otorhinolaryngology resident training. The combination of novel high-fidelity and low cost, practical models will ultimately maximize the resident's experience and training, making them better prepared and proficient when facing the live patient.

REFERENCES

1. Gallagher AG. VR to OR. In: Medicine meets virtual reality conference (MMVR 11). Newport Beach (CA); 2003.
2. Seymour NE, Gallagher AG, Roman SA, et al. Virtual reality training improves operating room performance: results of a randomized, double-blinded study. Ann Surg 2002;236(4):458–63 [discussion:463–4].
3. Caversaccio M, Eichenberger A, Hausler R. Virtual simulator as a training tool for endonasal surgery. Am J Rhinol 2003;17:283–90.
4. O'Toole RV, Playter RR, Krummel TM, et al. Measuring and developing suturing technique with a virtual reality surgical simulator. J Am Coll Surg 1999;189(1):114–27.

5. Satava RM. Virtual reality surgical simulator. The first steps. Surg Endosc 1993; 7(3):203–5.

6. Gorman PJ, Meier AH, Krummel TM. Computer-assisted training and learning in surgery. Comput Aided Surg 2000;5(2):120–30.

7. McGovern KT. Applications of virtual reality to surgery. BMJ 1994;308(6936): 1054–5.

8. Satava RM. Virtual endoscopy: diagnosis using 3-D visualization and virtual representation. Surg Endosc 1996;10(2):173–4.

9. Baillie J, Evangelou H, Jowel P, et al. The future of endoscopy simulation: a Duke perspective. Endoscopy 1992;24(Suppl 2):542–3.

10. Fried MP, Moharir VM, Sinmoto H, et al. Virtual laryngoscopy. Ann Otol Rhinol Laryngol 1999;108(3):221–6.

11. Peugnet F, Dubois P, Rouland JF. Virtual reality versus conventional training in retinal photocoagulation: a first clinical assessment. Comput Aided Surg 1998; 3(1):20–6.

12. Gladstone HB, Raugi GJ, Berg D, et al. Virtual reality for dermatologic surgery; virtually a reality in the 21st century. J Am Acad Dermatol 2000;42(1 Pt 1):106–12.

13. Berg D, Raugi G, Gladstone H, et al. Virtual reality simulators for dermatologic surgery: measuring their validity as a teaching tool. Dermatol Surg 2001;27(4): 370–4.

14. Oppenheimer P, Gupta A, Weghorst S, et al. The representation of blood flow in endourologic surgical simulations. Stud Health Technol Inform 2001;81:365–71.

15. Edmond CV Jr, Heskamp D, Sluis D, et al. ENT endoscopic surgical training simulator. Stud Health Technol Inform 1997;39:518–28.

16. Solyar A, Cuellar H, Sadoughi B, et al. Endoscopic sinus surgery simulator as a teaching tool for anatomy education. Am J Surg 2008;196:120–4.

17. Edmond CV Jr. Impact of the endoscopic sinus surgical simulator on operating room performance. Laryngoscope 2002;112(7 Pt 1):1148–58.

18. Rosen KR. The history of medical simulation. J Crit Care 2008;23:157–66.

19. Nogueira JF Jr, Nogueira Cruz D. Real models and virtual simulators in otolaryngology: review of literature. Braz J Otorhinolaryngol 2010;76(1):129–35.

20. Arora H, Uribe J, Ralph W, et al. Assessment of construct validity of the endoscopic sinus surgery simulator. Arch Otolaryngol Head Neck Surg 2005;131(3): 217–21.

21. Weit GJ, Stredney D, Wan D. Training and simulation in otolaryngology. Otolaryngol Clin North Am 2011;44:1333–50.

22. Gallagher AG, Ritter EM, Satava RM. Fundamental principles of validation, and reliability: rigorous science for the assessment of surgical education and training. Surg Endosc 2003;17(10):1525–9.

23. Hofstad EF, Vapenstad C, Chmarra MK, et al. A study of psychomotor skills in minimally invasive surgery: what differentiates expert and nonexpert performance. Surg Endosc 2013;27:854–63.

24. Gibber M, Kaye R, Fried MP. Virtual simulation in the surgical world. Otolaryngol Clin North Am 2009;42:891–900.

25. Fried MP, Satava R, Weghorst S, et al. The use of surgical simulators to reduce errors. In: Henriksen K, Battles JB, Marks ES, et al, editors. Advances in patient safety: from research to implementation. Rockville (MD): Agency for Healthcare Resesarch and Quality; 2005.

26. Fried MP, Satava R, Weghorst S, et al. Identifying and reducing errors with surgical simulation. Qual Saf Health Care 2004;13(Suppl 1):i19–26.

27. Fried MP, Sadoughi B, Gibber MJ, et al. From virtual reality to the operating room: the endoscopic sinus surgery simulator experiment. Otolaryngol Head Neck Surg 2010;142(2):202–7.
28. Weghorst S, Airola C, Oppenheimer P, et al. Validation of the Madigan ESS simulator. Stud Health Technol Inform 1998;50:399–405.
29. Rudman DT, Stredney D, Sessanna D, et al. Functional endoscopic sinus surgery training simulator. Laryngoscope 1998;10(8):1643–7.
30. Fried MP, Sadoughi B, Weghorst SJ, et al. Construct validity of the endoscopic sinus surgery simulator: II. Assessment of discriminant validity and expert benchmarking. Arch Otolaryngol Head Neck Surg 2007;133(4):350–7.
31. Uribe JI, Ralph WM Jr, Glaser AY, et al. Learning curves, acquisition, and retention of skills trained with the endoscopic sinus surgery simulator. Am J Rhinol 2004;18(2):87–92.
32. Fried MP, Kaye RJ, Gibber MJ, et al. Criterion-based (proficiency) training to improve surgical performance. Arch Otolaryngol Head Neck Surg 2012; 138(11):1024–9.
33. Tolsdorff B, Pommert A, Hohne KH, et al. Virtual reality: a new paranasal sinus surgery simulator. Laryngoscope 2010;120:420–6.
34. Varshney R, Frenkiel S, Nguyen LH, et al. The McGill simulator for endoscopic sinus surgery (MSESS): a validation study. J Otolaryngol Head Neck Surg 2014;43:40.
35. Varshney R, Frenkiel S, Nguyen LH, et al. Development of the McGill simulator for endoscopic sinus surgery: a new high-fidelity virtual reality simulator for endoscopic sinus surgery. Am J Rhinol Allergy 2014;28(4):330–4.
36. Fortes B, Balsalobre L, Weber R, et al. Endoscopic sinus surgery dissection courses using a real simulator: the benefits of this training. Braz J Otorhinolaryngol 2016;82:26–32.
37. Malekzadeh S, Pfisterer MJ, Wilson B, et al. A novel low-cost sinus surgery task trainer. Otolaryngol Head Neck Surg 2011;145(4):530–3.
38. Wais M, Ooi E, Vescan AD, et al. The effect of low-fidelity endoscopic sinus surgery simulators on surgical skill. Int Forum Allergy Rhinol 2012;2(1):20–6.

Simulators for Laryngeal and Airway Surgery

James A. Burns, MD[a],*, Lacey K. Adkins, MD[a], Seth Dailey, MD[b], Adam M. Klein, MD[c]

KEYWORDS

- Simulation • Larynx • Airway • Microlaryngoscopy • Virtual reality

KEY POINTS

- Simulators for laryngeal and airway surgery have become increasingly important in residency training.
- Effective laryngeal and airway surgery simulators can be made from low-cost and easily attainable materials.
- Simulators should be able to measure a subject's performance, and feedback from trainees is an important part of developing useful laryngeal and airway surgery simulators.

INTRODUCTION

Laryngeal and airway surgery require precise technique and a significant amount of mastered skill that can be difficult to obtain during otolaryngology residency training. Traditional on-the-job training with mentor oversight has become more challenging because of time and fiscal constraints, a growing medicolegal environment, and higher patient expectations and awareness of receiving care in an academic training environment. Procedural simulators have become increasingly important in residency training (eg, temporal bone simulators, bronchoscopy simulators, cadaver dissection courses), and in new-surgeon skill acquisition (eg, transoral robotic surgery, photoangiolytic laser laryngeal surgery). Current otolaryngology residency program requirements mandate that residents "must demonstrate knowledge of anatomy through procedural skills demonstrated in cadaver dissection, temporal bone lab, and/or simulation labs." Nevertheless, in a survey by Shah and colleagues,[1] only 18.8% of US otolaryngology residents were very satisfied with their phonomicrosurgery experience

The authors have nothing to disclose.

[a] Center for Laryngeal Surgery and Voice Rehabilitation, Massachusetts General Hospital, One Bowdoin Square, 11th Floor, Boston, MA 02114, USA; [b] Division of Otolaryngology, Department of Surgery, University of Wisconsin School of Medicine and Public Health, 750 Highland Avenue, Madison, WI 53705, USA; [c] Department of Otolaryngology–Head and Neck Surgery, Emory Voice Center, Emory University School of Medicine, 550 Peachtree Street, Northeast, 9th Floor, Suite 4400, Atlanta, GA 30308, USA
* Corresponding author.
E-mail address: burns.james@mgh.harvard.edu

Otolaryngol Clin N Am 50 (2017) 903–922
http://dx.doi.org/10.1016/j.otc.2017.05.003
0030-6665/17/© 2017 Elsevier Inc. All rights reserved.

oto.theclinics.com

in residency. More than 87% thought they would benefit from laboratory-based training.

Simulators are particularly useful for developing skills in laryngeal and airway surgery. These surgeries are often performed by a single operator and therefore do not lend themselves well to a more traditional mentor relationship where the teacher assists the trainee. In-office laryngeal and airway procedures present additional challenges in awake patients, whose anxiety about a procedure and strong desire for success may preclude their willingness to participate in procedural skill training. Mandates for increased patient safety and more uniform training curricula have spurred the development of physical training platforms that allow learners to emulate teaching models such as the temporal bone drilling station that has now become a mandatory part of Accreditation Council for Graduate Medical Education accreditation of Otolaryngology-Head and Neck surgery resident training programs. In these models, experts mentor trainees in a zero-risk environment where laryngeal and airway surgeries as well as office-based procedures are simulated on cadaveric animal structures, human larynges, or trainers that incorporate noncadaveric materials.

This article reviews the literature pertaining to simulators and ex vivo training methods used in teaching laryngeal and airway surgery and highlights the efficacy of these models. Descriptions of simulators reported for use in microlaryngoscopy, transcervical laryngeal injection, bronchoscopy, intubation, flexible laryngoscopy, cricothyroidotomy, and tracheotomy are presented.

PHONOSURGERY TRAINER AND ASSESSMENT OF SKILL ACQUISITION

The laryngeal dissection station originally developed by Dailey and colleagues[2] was made from cheap materials and allowed for a physical platform onto which a human or animal cadaveric larynx could be mounted (**Figs. 1–4**). Both endoscopic and open surgery could be simulated with instrumentation identical to the operating room. A focus on the preservation of tissue for maximum utility of larynges, sometimes hard to come by, was maintained. Again mirroring the temporal bone experience, dissection manuals by Johns and Klein and then by Dailey and Verma helped to provide learners with detailed step-by-step surgical directions with emphasis on clinical pearls and pitfalls of the various procedures.[3–5] Implementation of this type of training into resident training programs was demonstrated later by Verma, including cost analysis for dissemination and implementation of laryngeal training.[4] With cost always an issue, Verma then developed a low-cost version of the dissection station able to reliably be constructed with easy-to-find materials.[6] This station was termed the versatile optimally constructed aid for laryngeal surgery simulation (**Fig. 5**). Less than $100, it is now being used across the United States. With the beginnings of a more standardized training curriculum under way, additional refinements were now possible to mirror surgical precision for task-specific evaluation as seen in laparoscopic training in general surgery.

It is well known that endoscopic surgery involving tissue manipulation for so-called benign lesions of the vocal fold (eg, polyps, cysts, nodules) is extremely challenging. Surgeons must work through a small-bore laryngoscope while using long fulcrum arm instruments to maximally preserve the delicate layered structure of the lamina propria. They must preserve overlying epithelium to prevent healing by secondary intention and subsequent scar formation, all this in a setting of looking through a binocular microscope and maintaining adequate ergonomics to prevent muscle fatigue with subsequent loss of instrument stability and accuracy. This set of circumstances where mistakes can lead to poor phonatory outcomes is ideal

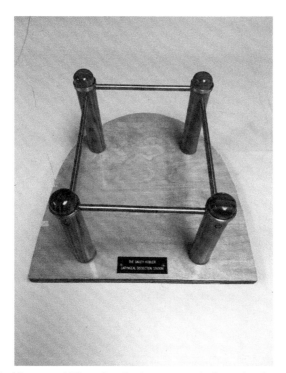

Fig. 1. The original Laryngeal Dissection Station was made from simple construction materials. A wide base was designed for stability.

for evaluation of instrument control. Therefore, a magnetic tracking device was explored for phonomicrosurgical evaluations where the motion of the tips of the instruments could be tracked in 3 dimensions with high-level time resolution.[7] Three experts and 6 novices were tested using a standardized phonomicrosurgical task. Experts demonstrated significantly better motion smoothness for the dominant hand. For the nondominant hand, experts demonstrated better motion smoothness, shorter path length, and better depth perception. Experts also demonstrated higher quality of operation based on subjective observation of the final result. No significant difference in time was noted in completion of the task between experts and novices.

Experience with the magnetic motion tracking device led to the evaluation of how different operative situations affect instrument motion. For example, it was hypothesized that a head-mounted microscope might improve performance parameters in phonomicrosurgery.[8] Again, the motion tracking device was used along with additional cumulative summation analysis assessment to track the quality of the operation, the time to completion, as well as specific motion parameters such as "smoothness" (**Fig. 6**). The motion parameters from the head-mounted microscope were significantly better than the standing microscope. However, the time to completion was longer than that from the standing microscope, and the subjective quality of performance of the task was worse. Interestingly, the data did not support adaptation of the learners to the head-mounted microscope. To date, one additional hypothesis has been tested using the head-mounted microscope. It is hypothesized that supporting the arms of a surgeon who is performing phonomicrosurgery will offer better instrument control than

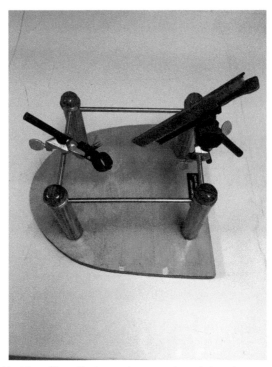

Fig. 2. A laryngeal holder affixes the larynx in space. A prototype laryngeal speculum allows for simulation of endoscopic surgery.

a surgeon who does not have arm support. By using the motion tracking device on the ends of phonomicrosurgical instruments, different conditions of no arm support, elbow support, and forearm support were tested for the standard phonomicrosurgical task (**Fig. 7**).[9] It was found that with forearm support, the nondominant hand showed improved smoothness, improved distance traveled, and a shorter pathway to the target than no arm support. There was also improved motion control in the dominant hand with elbow support. Elbow support resulted in increased steadiness, shorter surgical path, and better distance traveled. Better operation quality was associated with increased motion control in the nondominant hand. It appears that surgical ergonomics seem to matter when fine motor tasks are performed in phonomicrosurgery, further underscoring the importance of simulation in teaching laryngeal and airway surgical skills.

CADAVERIC LARYNGES AND LOW-FIDELITY TRAINERS

Although the use of cadaveric tissue for medical education and training began in 500 BC,[10] its application for the purpose of phonomicrosurgical training began in the 1960s when the first phonomicrosurgical instruments were introduced by Jako.[11] In recent decades, working with cadaveric larynges in the laboratory setting has become more difficult. Obtaining larynges can be challenging, and an infrastructure is necessary for their proper storage and disposal. It can also be difficult to physically set them up and reliably establish and maintain exposure of the vocal folds while training. The layered microstructure of the vocal fold is typically abnormal in

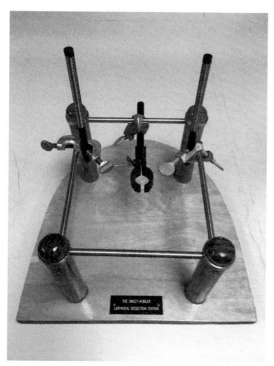

Fig. 3. The lateral bars hold vertical bars to which sutures can be placed from the cadaveric larynx for stability.

texture because of preservation methods of freezing or formalin fixation; thus, the benefit of real soft tissue is diminished. Cadaveric larynges are good for single use only, and finally, there is rarely any abnormality on which to practice phonomicrosurgical resection techniques. Porcine and bovine larynges are suitable and affordable alternatives; however, they are still previously frozen tissue and share the disadvantages of human tissue in terms of texture. Thus, if each trainee wishes to practice a procedure several times, then large and/or frequent orders must be placed. These reasons have provided, in part, the impetus for the development of synthetic phonomicrosurgical trainers.

The support apparatuses, or modules, available for cadaveric laryngeal dissection often have drawbacks as well. Some are too cumbersome for use in the laboratory setting, whereas others are not conducive to quick and reliable laryngeal exposure. The ones that do offer certain features and excellent degrees of freedom to optimize exposure still lack wrist supports to allow surgical trainees to hone their skills in an ideal ergonomic setting.[12–15] Phonomicrosurgical training devices should simulate the surgical experience as much as possible; thus, the entire apparatus needs to be designed with that function in mind.

In an effort to address these issues, several low-fidelity phonomicrosurgical simulators have been developed.[12,14–16] Contag and colleagues[16] described a low-cost laryngeal dissection module (LDM) that consisted of a laryngoscope station (Dailey and colleagues)[2] and a model larynx with tissue paper vocal folds. The LDM allowed residents and medical students to practice and improve their phonomicrosurgical skills under mentorship without any untoward consequences to a patient.

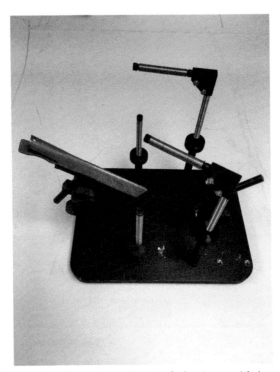

Fig. 4. A second-generation device is made out of aluminum with interchangeable parts and easy-to-clean surfaces.

HIGH-FIDELITY TRAINERS

Although the LDM and other trainers offer much in the way of phonomicrosurgical simulation, there are 2 main limitations: (1) the lack of similarity to the microstructured architecture of the true vocal fold with an imbedded lesion, and (2) the poor ergonomic similarity to the operative experience. To that end, a high-fidelity trainer that is more consistent with a true phonomicrosurgical experience offers advantages over an LDM. High-fidelity trainers contain materials with better rheological properties that emulate the various layers and consistency of human vocal folds and contain a synthetic "phonotraumatic lesion" integrated into each fold beneath the "epithelium." A larynx scaffold that opens in the midline sagittal plane allows for the insertion and removal of the synthetic vocal folds (**Figs. 8** and **9**). The new support module was designed to optimize operative ergonomics with an adjustable laryngoscope and wrist supports (**Figs. 10** and **11**). This phonomicrosurgical trainer, as well as others, has objectively quantified technical errors and facilitated training to improve phonomicrosurgical skills and is becoming an important tool in residency training.

As surgical simulators continue to gain traction and credibility in the new model of surgical education that is linked to the quality movement in health care, we are likely looking toward a future of case-specific simulation. The utilization of computer technology, such as virtual reality,[17,18] will allow a surgeon to upload a case and "rehearse" a surgery before the "final performance." New devices, such as 3D printers,[19,20] are already being used to create readily available, realistic, reusable, and low-cost

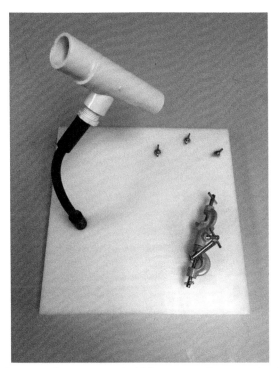

Fig. 5. The Versatile Optimally Constructed Aid for Laryngeal Surgery Simulation (VOCALSS). Low-cost parts that are commercially manufactured and easily assembled make self-production more available for less than $100.

anatomic models that provide haptic feedback for skills training. Technological advances need to be applied in order to fully optimize the learning potential of budding laryngeal surgeons to objectively gauge their operative skills and functional outcomes through simulation.

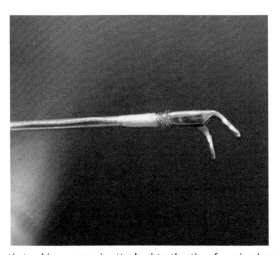

Fig. 6. The magnetic tracking sensor is attached to the tip of a microlaryngeal forceps.

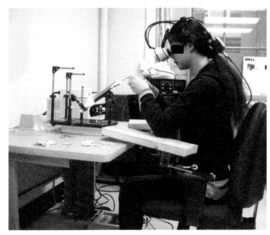

Fig. 7. The head-mounted microscope is worn by a study participant demonstrating how it is used for phonomicrosurgery.

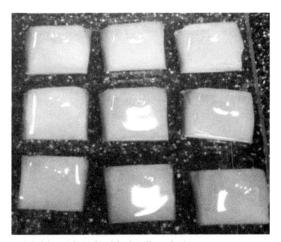

Fig. 8. Synthetic vocal folds with imbedded yellow lesions.

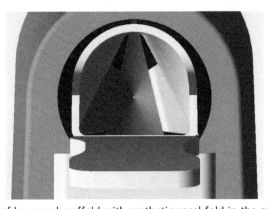

Fig. 9. Schematic of laryngeal scaffold with synthetic vocal fold in the anatomic position.

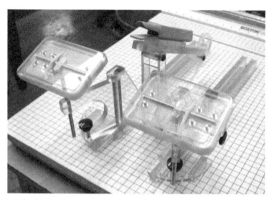

Fig. 10. Module with built-in laryngoscope and wrist rests.

MICROLARYNGOSCOPY SIMULATORS

1. Holliday and colleagues[12] published a validation study for a low-cost simulator where 16 attending otolaryngologists performed 3 separate skill-based tasks. The simulator consisted of a 1.25-inch polyvinyl chloride (PVC) pipe cut in 12-inch lengths and fit to a plywood base with conduit hangers and copper pipes. The PVC pipes were then notched to accommodate a Kantor-Berci laryngoscope on one end and inter-changeable laryngeal cartridges at the opposite end. The cartridges were made from 1.25-inch-diameter plastic pipe with 3 notches cut in the end, allowing rubber bands to be looped around them to represent vocal folds (**Fig. 12**). Self-sealing plastic wrap was used as epithelium, and bacitracin ointment was injected to simulate Reinke space. Three basic microlaryngoscopy tasks were then performed as 3 different modules.

The first basic module consisted of 3 sutures passed through the rubber band. Two sutures were held in place by friction, and the third was knotted. The task consisted of grasping and removing each suture, cutting the last one. The second module repre-sented an epithelial lesion. For this, silicone-based caulk was applied to the plastic wrap along the medial edge. For the task, a 24-g laryngeal needle was used to inject an air bubble (representing subepithelial injection) to form a plane of dissection. The lesion was then grasped and excised with microscissors. On the same cartridge, the opposite vocal fold rubber band had a 5-0 silk suture sewn 3 times through the band and tied with an air knot to simulate a subepithelial lesion. After the subepithelial

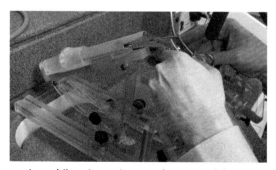

Fig. 11. Subject operating while using wrist rests; larynx model mounted in module.

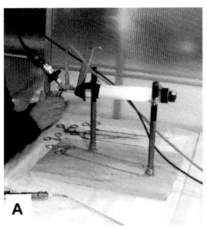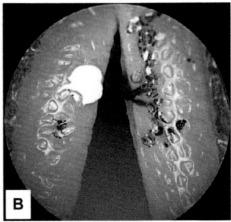

Fig. 12. (*A*) Simulation model and stand. (*B*) Endoscopic view of epithelial (*left cord*) and subepithelial (*right cord*) lesion task.

injection of air, the person would create a microflap, dissect the lesion free and cut the suture, and then redrape the flap. The third module represented papilloma, consisting of plastic wrap stretched across the cartridge, followed by grapefruit, then another sheet of plastic wrap. The task consisted of incising the wrap in a cruciate fashion and debulking the papilloma with a microdebrider until the deep plastic wrap was revealed.

Attending-level laryngologists were then given a questionnaire regarding the value of each exercise. Of the respondents, 100% agreed that the basic skills and epithelial lesion exercises were valuable; 88% agreed that the subepithelial lesion exercise was valuable, and 86% agreed that the papilloma module was valuable. All of the attendings agreed that the simulator helped to develop phonomicrosurgical dexterity and skills related to microsurgery.[12]

2. Nixon and colleagues[15] described a hybrid simulator, placing a porcine larynx within an airway training mannequin. The mannequin had realistic anatomy of teeth, tongue, palate, and other upper airway structures. They performed a lateral pharyngotomy within the plastic laryngopharynx, placing the porcine larynx within and allowing the plastic to hold it in place using Velcro to reapproximate the pharyngotomy. They then demonstrated that suspension microlaryngoscopy could be performed with the simulator.

3. Awad and colleagues[21] used Yorkshire porcine larynxes mounted within a cardboard cup and fixed to a work top. Five tasks were done: examination under anesthesia, vocal cord biopsy of a marked lesion, medialization injection, submucosal flap elevation, and posterior cordotomy. Participants responded to a 20-point Likert scale, and results showed that participants thought this was a suitable task trainer for 4 of the 5 tasks. The exception was the posterior cordotomy task, because less than 75% thought it was useful because it was performed with cold steel instead of laser.[21]

4. Fleming and colleagues[14] created an operating room immersive microlaryngoscopy simulator. They recruited 15 participants; 9 were classified as novice (less than 50 microlaryngoscopy performed) and 6 were experienced. They used an ear, nose, and throat (ENT) operating microscope with a 400-mm lens, a suspension laryngoscope, and the laryngeal model that consisted of a synthetic vocal cord model

inserted into an airway mannequin. Each session lasted up to 10 minutes. The laryngoscope had to be inserted and suspended, and the microscope positioned and focused. The task itself involved dissecting a polypoid lesion from the superficial layer of the vocal fold.

On a 5-point Likert scale, the simulator scored a 4 and a 4.07 for realism and fair assessment of skills. The Checklist Assessment for Microlaryngeal Surgery (CAMS) and Global Rating Assessment for Microlaryngeal Surgery (GRAMS) were compared between the advanced and novice groups. The average marks of the novice group compared with the experienced group for CAMS was significantly different, however not significantly different for the GRAMS assessment.[14]

5. Zambricki and colleagues[22] describe a grape-based model for phonomicrosurgery. They mounted a laryngoscope on a stand constructed from 1-inch PVC tubing, stabilizing the barrel with silicone injected into a cross-connector around the plastic-wrapped laryngoscope barrel. The tissue model consisted of grapes imbedded within gelatin placed in a pet food dish. Each grape was marked with a 1-cm line at the midline. Residents were then asked to position the microscope, make an incision through the grape skin along the line, and elevate bilateral grape skin "subepithelial" flaps. They then trimmed a crescent from each flap and simulated vocal fold medialization injection by injecting mayonnaise through an injection needle. Each of the 30 residents and fellows were given a pretest session followed by 20 minutes of independent practice before a posttest session. The videos of their sessions were deidentified and graded by a laryngologist on a 3-point scale for various items, including microscope positioning, incision creation, flap elevation, preservation of remaining tissue, and total time required. They looked at 30 residents and fellows, showing significant improvements across all variables from the pretest to posttest. Senior residents performed better on positioning the microscope, preserving remaining tissue, and taking less time to complete the tasks. There was no difference between junior and senior residents on their ratings for incisions, elevation of flaps, or excision of tissue. All residents reported improved comfort with microlaryngeal instrumentation after the simulation session.[23]

CHORIOALLANTOIC MEMBRANE MODEL FOR PHOTOANGIOLYSIS

Recently, there have been evolving photoangiolytic laser techniques for the treatment of laryngeal abnormality.[23–25] These abnormalities (recurrent respiratory papillomatosis, dysplasia, selected cancers, and limited phonotraumatic vascular lesions) are often associated with aberrant microcirculation, which makes them effectively treated with photoangiolytic lasers. Angiolytic lasers (Potassium-titanyl-phosphate [KTP], Pulsed dye laser [PDL]) involute the microcirculation because the laser energy is more selectively absorbed by hemoglobin. The focused energy leads to intravascular photocoagulation and vessel ablation. With this emerging technology, there is a need to equip treating surgeons with the basic science and clinical experience to enable safe widespread application of the technology in laryngeal surgery. The chorioallantoic membrane (CAM) model provides an excellent bench-top simulation of the true vocal fold superficial lamina propria with its microcirculation. The CAM is a vascular membrane of a developing chick embryo and thus provides a perfusing model to study the effects of lasers on microcirculation (**Fig. 13**).[26]

The CAM was reported more than 70 years ago[27] and recently used as a model for laser research.[28] However, this model has remarkable similarities to the superficial lamina propria, which facilitates simulation of selected phonomicrosurgical skills. There is an array of small vessels in the CAM ranging from the equivalent of human capillaries to larger vessels simulating vocal-fold varices (see **Fig. 13**). The CAM

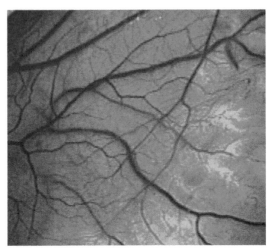

Fig. 13. A magnified view of the chick CAM microcirculation suspended within the albumen that simulates microvasculature of human vocal folds.

vessels are suspended within the albumen in a manner similar to the microcirculation of the superficial lamina propria on the human true vocal fold. Thus, the CAM is an ideal model with which to study laser coagulation and heat effects and to practice photoangiolytic surgical skills.

Using the CAM model with photoangiolytic lasers, the surgeon can simulate the working environment for selected laryngeal vascular lesions at minimal cost. The nuances of these lasers and their delivery systems (ie, fiber size) along with different settings (power, pulse width, and so forth) and fiber-to-tissue distance can be safely analyzed while achieving an appropriate comfort level using this technology. Benchtop use of angiolytic lasers with a stereoscopic microscope and the CAM will familiarize surgeons with the intricacies of the pulsed KTP laser and PDL with 3-dimensional high magnification. This experience is especially valuable for surgeons who have purchased an angiolytic laser for office-based surgery (2-dimensional imaging and a moving microcirculatory target) and who will not have the benefit of observational learning in the operating room under general anesthesia. Taken together, the CAM model facilitates effective safe translation of fiber-based photoangiolytic laser skills to clinical settings in laryngeal surgery.[26]

TRANSCERVICAL INJECTION MODEL

Manual skill acquisition for performing transcervical laryngeal injections is not often prioritized during otolaryngology training. Providing procedural instruction and training for residents and fellows to perform transcervical laryngeal injections can be challenging, especially in the era of restricted resident work hours. The inherent difficulty in teaching a technique that relies on tactile and auditory feedback in awake and often anxious patients, combined with a limited number of opportunities during clinical training, creates a need for a simulation model to increase the otolaryngologist's confidence with the procedure. A transcervical laryngeal injection simulation model was developed that provides real-time auditory feedback to determine that the needle has been placed properly within specific laryngeal muscles.[29] Realistic tactile feedback is achieved by creating a rigid laryngeal framework that simulates the cartilaginous framework suspended in silicone, which simulates the soft tissues of the neck. The auditory feedback simulates electromyography (EMG) guidance during transcervical injection (**Fig. 14**). The system uses needles identical to those used for transcervical botulinum toxin injection. Presimulation and postsimulation question-naires asked respondents to rate their comfort with the procedure, and their study re-ported a significant improvement in the comfort of respondents' postsimulation training. Results demonstrated significantly improved confidence levels for otolaryn-gology residents performing transcervical thyroarytenoid muscle injections after using the model. Most residents had obtained little or no training in transcervical laryngeal injections in their residency, with nearly all indicating that they would like to receive more procedural instruction.

LARYNGEAL INJECTION SIMULATORS

1. Cabrera-Muffly and colleagues[30] made a low-cost transcervical laryngeal injection trainer. They used a toilet paper roll with a long thin balloon inserted through it to look like vocal folds. Cardboard was placed on the roll to act as the thyroid cartilage, and a zip tie was used as the cricoid ring. They added batting and cloth to simulate over-lying tissue so that residents had to palpate for landmarks. Each model cost about $1 and, because they had 2 vocal folds, could be used for 2 injections. Residents received a handout with instruction to practice vocal fold injection and then per-formed the injection using thinned yogurt. Each resident also completed a presimu-lation and postsimulation survey. There was no change in perceived confidence before and after the simulation. However, residents stated that the simulator would help to improve their confidence and was a good method of learning. All of the res-idents would recommend the simulation to others. Also, although no specific tech-nique was advocated, the residents performed both transcricothyroid and transthyrohyoid techniques.[30]

2. Amin and colleagues[31] described a hands-on trainer that used fresh cadaver larynges to simulate peroral injection techniques. For suspension microlaryngoscopy

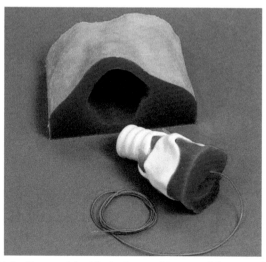

Fig. 14. Laryngeal injection model with the internal laryngeal framework and neck soft tis-sue mold.

simulation, they created a larynx holder that would allow the larynx to be fixed with suture at the distal end of a laryngoscope. Then, a 0° endoscopic rod or a microscope could be used to complete the simulation. For a peroral technique, they used an intubation mannequin with a patent upper airway. They subsequently removed the mannequin's larynx and placed a cadaver larynx in the neck. A chip-tip endoscope was then passed through the mannequin's nose and projected onto a monitor. The trainees completed a presimulation and postsimulation questionnaire comparing their comfort level on an analogue scale of 0 to 100. A total of 22 trainees completed the survey, and their comfort level improved from 22 to 52 for peroral vocal fold injection and 69 to 85 for microlaryngoscopy vocal fold injection. It was thought that the greater improvement in confidence experienced with the peroral injection was because most of the participants had no prior experience with this technique.[31]

BRONCHOSCOPY
Flexible

1. Colt and colleagues[32] looked at virtual reality programs for flexible bronchoscopy. They underwent 2 hours of direct teaching, 2 hours of supervised practice using the simulator, and up to 4 hours of individual unsupervised practice. The virtual reality skill center had a proxy flexible bronchoscope, a robotic interface to track the motions and reproduce all forces felt during an examination, and a monitor to display computer-generated images. The virtual patient would breathe, cough, bleed, and have change in vital signs. It also records the duration of the procedure, the amount of topical anesthetic used, the number and sequence of bronchial segments examined, and the number of collisions. These 5 subjects were then compared with 4 pulmonologists who had performed more than 200 flexible bronchoscopies. At the end of their 8 hours of practice, subjects would perform a thorough bronchoscopic examination on an inanimate bronchoscopy model and were graded by 2 pulmonologists. Novice trainers missed fewer segments after training and had fewer contacts. However, there was no change in speed. There was no statistically significant difference between novice scores after training and skilled physician scores.[32]

2. Blum and colleagues[33] looked at surgical residents using the same virtual reality bronchoscopy simulator described above. They compared interns to PGY2 or PGY3 residents. Residents that were assigned to the simulator were allowed to practice for as long as they wanted. They were then timed as they performed an intraoperative bronchoscopy and were instructed to examine every segment. The number of times bronchi were redundantly explored was also recorded. The examiner and the subject then evaluated the level of confidence and proficiency on a scale of 0 to 5. The time to completion was no different between groups; however, the simulator group required less verbal direction. The simulator groups' examinations were as complete as the experienced group, but they were rated as less confident.[33]

Rigid

1. Salud and colleagues[34] used a commercially available bronchoscopy model and fixed it with sensors to detect possible abrasions for a rigid bronchoscope. The sensors were placed along the tongue, hypopharynx, vocal folds, tracheoesophageal junction, and anterior trachea. They tested 38 people: 14 experts and 24 novices (as they rated themselves). There was no significant difference in the amount of time to complete a rigid bronchoscopy; however, the number of abrasions was higher among novices (3.37 vs 2.93) but not statistically significant.[34]

Foreign Body Retrieval

1. Deutsch and colleagues[35] used high-fidelity mannequins to simulate aerodigestive foreign bodies. Their model would initially demonstrate retractions and asymmetric breath sounds. It would then develop hypoxia and cyanosis. With laryngeal instrumentation, it would develop laryngospasm, requiring positive pressure ventilation. A foreign body was visualized in the left main bronchus and was grasped with an optical forceps. On being withdrawn, it would be stripped from the forceps in the subglottis, requiring another removal.[35]

2. Deutsch and colleagues[36] published another study with the above mannequin, looking at 8 residents and 1 pediatric ENT fellow. They included a foreign body injection by placing a coin in the esophageal introitus. Each exercise was repeated until trained to competence. Participants worked in teams of 2 (a junior and senior resident) or 3 (plus a fellow). They then answered a questionnaire based on a 5-point Likert scale. The highest ratings were for training cognitive and psychomotor endoscopy skills (4.89), preventing and managing complications (4.67), and team process (4.78).[36]

INTUBATION/FLEXIBLE FIBEROPTIC LARYNGOSCOPY

1. Deutschmann and colleagues[37] simulated transnasal flexible fiberoptic laryngoscopy with 68 medical students and junior residents. Subjects observed an endoscopy being performed by the attending and received instruction on how to operate the endoscope. They then performed an endoscopy on a patient. Afterward, they were randomized to the nonsimulation group or the simulation group, with the simulation group using a low-fidelity simulator consisting of a flexible endoscope and a hollow ball with multiple fenestrations inside a glove. They would practice going in and out of the fenestrations for 45 minutes. Afterward, both groups would return to clinic to perform another endoscopy on a patient. They analyzed the time to glottis visualization, the percentage of time of adequate airway visualization, and the total number of mucosal collisions. The senior author and the patients also subjectively evaluated them on a 10-point scale for patient comfort, ease of manipulation, and learner comfort. Both the simulation and the nonsimulation group experienced improvement in the time to glottis visualization and mucosal contacts. Both groups also demonstrated more comfort and better manipulation between the first and second endoscopies, whereas patient comfort did not change. However, there was no difference between the simulation and nonsimulation group. In fact, when the results were stratified by the number of endoscopies performed, results suggested that the simulation group, beyond repeated endoscopy, showed no benefit.[37]

2. There is something to be said for repetition. Laeeq and colleagues[38] specifically looked at the number of endoscopies it took before a person became competent by evaluating 15 medical students. Each student had instruction and demonstration by an attending and then were allowed to practice on a mannequin. Each attempt was graded by an attending, and students were allowed to keep practicing until they were deemed competent by the attending on 2 consecutive attempts. An average of 6 attempts was required for the medical students to become competent.[38]

3. De Oliveira and colleagues[39] designed a virtual reality application (iLarynx) that used the built-in accelerometer of an iPhone. The accelerometers could duplicate the twisting of a scope with the left thumb controlling the tip deflection and the right thumb advancing the endoscope to simulate fiberoptic intubation. Medical students were given a lecture on airway anatomy and intubation technique before being assigned to further simulation or no further training. The iLarynx group was allowed

30 minutes for practice. Afterward, all of the participants performed transoral fiberoptic intubation on a simulation mannequin (AirSim) a total of 10 consecutive times to view the carina. The primary measurement was the amount of time it took for them to visualize the carina. If they took more than 120 seconds, the attempt was viewed as failed. They were also graded on a 5-point scale on their scope manipulation ability. In total, there were 24 failed attempts in the standard group and 4 in the iLarynx group. The time to carina visualization was also lower in the iLarynx group; however, there was no difference in the skills checklist or global assessment score between the 2 groups.[39]

CRICOTHYROTOMY/TRACHEOTOMY
Cricothyrotomy

1. Aho and colleagues[40] describe a low-fidelity model for teaching a cricothyrotomy. They constructed a model out of a toilet paper roll to simulate the trachea and larynx, Styrofoam tubing to simulate overlying soft tissue, fabric for the skin, cardboard for the thyroid cartilage, and a zip tie as the cricoid ring. Fifty-four trainees were then evaluated based upon a procedural checklist derived from consensus on proper emergency cricothyrotomy technique by 6 staff general surgeons. The checklist included a generous midline incision, bluntly spreading in the midline, exposing the cricothyroid membrane, bluntly perforating the membrane, spreading the membrane with a clamp, keeping the clamp open, inserting the endotracheal tube, twisting the endotracheal tube in place, blowing up the cuff and connecting to oxygen, checking CO_2, and securing the tube. The trainees consisted of medical students, surgical interns, and PGY-3 general surgery residents. As would be expected, the scores varied significantly across the groups, with medical students scoring 1.8, interns scoring 3.5, and residents scoring 4.9. Each model was estimated to cost less than 10 cents and was graded by the trainees as educational.[40] The low cost of the study was emphasized, citing the Wong and colleagues[41] study that showed at least 5 attempts on mannequins were needed before residents could perform cricothyroidotomy in 40 seconds.

2. Friedman and colleagues[42] compared the utility of high- and low-fidelity models in teaching cricothyrotomy. They used 22 anesthesia residents who had never performed one before, and they all performed a pretest cricothyrotomy on a cadaver where only their hands were recorded and graded by a blinded grader. They were then randomized to perform 2 simulations on a high-fidelity Sim-Man with an anatomically correct larynx and whose skin and cricothyroidotomy membrane were replaced after each use of a low-fidelity model. The low-fidelity model consisted of airway tubing where a notch was cut out and covered in tape to simulate the cricothyroid membrane covered in a silicon membrane to simulate skin. Within 2 weeks of simulation, the residents performed a posttest on human cadavers. There was no statistical difference in the change from pretest to posttest scores for those who used the low-fidelity vs those who used the high-fidelity model. Both groups showed significant improvement in their performance and a decrease in the time it took to perform the procedure.[42]

3. Proctor and colleagues[43] compared a haptic-enabled virtual reality simulation vs mannequin simulator for cricothyrotomy. The mannequin used was a HapMed mannequin, which allowed for ventilation, palpation of the cricothyroid membrane, and bleeding. CricSim was a virtual human that would operate on a desktop PC with 3-dimensional glasses and 2 haptic interface devises. Thirty-two combat medics then used both simulations after being randomized to the order in which they were

performed. They then examined user recommendations afterward, with 88.46% recommending the CricSim and 92.3% recommending the HapMed. The CricSim trended toward having a clearer and more understandable visual interaction as well as being easier to learn to operate. However, the CricSim and HapMed were equivalent in ease to become skillful, tactile interactions, and force feedback.[43]

4. Jayaraman and colleagues[44] compared a standard lecture to general surgery residents on cricothyroidotomy to a lecture plus simulation. Before instruction, the residents completed assessments of self-efficacy and knowledge. Those assigned to the simulation group used a Laerdal simulation torso with replaceable cricothyroid membrane and neck skin for approximately 10 minutes. Later that afternoon, both groups were evaluated on their performance on porcine models. Afterward, although there was no difference in self-reported self-efficacy or knowledge, the simulation group did have higher laboratory scores indicating better performance and took less time to complete the cricothyroidotomy (5.87 vs 9.89 minutes).[44]

Percutaneous Tracheotomy

1. Gardiner and colleagues[45] describe an animal model to help simulate endoscopic-guided percutaneous tracheostomy. A pig thorax laid on its back with the head extended was intubated orally and attached to a ventilator. The fiberoptic bronchoscope was attached to a television camera and monitor and used to practice both the Ciaglia dilatational technique and the Portex forceps technique, slowly making successive tracheostomy sites working up from the sternal notch so each animal could have multiple uses.

The bronchoscope was first inserted and the bronchial anatomy explored before it was pulled back to lie within the trachea. The area of insertion was palpated and confirmed endoscopically, and then a skin incision was made. Using Bougie dilators or forceps, the fistula was created within the trachea with the bronchoscope being used to confirm placement and make sure the posterior tracheal wall was not damaged. The tracheotomy was then placed and confirmed endoscopically and a tracheobronchoscopy was performed. Twenty trainees rated the model as useful in learning the techniques, but no further statistical comparison was made between those that used the simulator and those that did not.[45]

SUMMARY

Laryngeal and airway surgery require precise technique and significant mastered skill that can be difficult to obtain during otolaryngology residency training. Simulators are particularly useful for developing laryngeal and airway surgery skills that will ultimately be evaluated in a competency-based manner. Simulators reported for use in microlaryngoscopy can be high fidelity or low fidelity and can be extremely inexpensive while still effective. Simulators for laryngeal injections, bronchoscopy, intubation, flexible laryngoscopy, cricothyroidotomy, and tracheotomy are available for obtaining and maintaining these skills. Assessing the usefulness of laryngeal and airway simulators is an important part of incorporating them into training programs.

REFERENCES

1. Shah MD, Johns MM 3rd, Statham M, et al. Assessment of phonomicrosurgical training in otolaryngology residencies: a resident survey. Laryngoscope 2013; 123(6):1474–7.
2. Dailey SH, Kobler JB, Zeitels SM. A laryngeal dissection station: educational paradigms in phonosurgery. Laryngoscope 2004;114(5):878–82.

3. Dailey SH, Verma SP. Laryngeal dissection and surgery guide. New York: Thieme; 2013.

4. Klein AM, Johns MM. Laryngeal dissection and phonosurgical atlas. San Diego: Plural; 2009.

5. Verma SP, Dailey SH, McMurray JS, et al. Implementation of a program for surgical education in laryngology. Laryngoscope 2010;120(11):2241–6.

6. Foulad A, Bui P, Dailey SH, et al. VOCALSS: versatile optimally constructed aid for laryngeal surgery simulation. Laryngoscope 2015;125(5):1169–71.

7. Chen T, Surender K, Vamos AC, et al. Quantitative evaluation of phonomicrosurgical manipulations using a magnetic motion tracking system. Laryngoscope 2014;124(9):2107–13.

8. Chen T, Vamos AC, Dailey SH, et al. CUSUM analysis of learning curves for the head-mounted microscope in phonomicrosurgery. Laryngoscope 2016;126(10): 2295–300.

9. Chen T, Vamos AC, Dailey SH, et al. A study of phonomicrosurgical arm support postures using a magnetic motion tracking system. Laryngoscope 2016;126(4): 918–22.

10. Okada DM, Sousa AM, Huertas RA, et al. Surgical simulator for temporal bone dissection training. Braz J Otorhinolaryngol 2010;76(5):575–8.

11. Zeitels SM. Premalignant epithelium and microinvasive cancer of the vocal fold: the evolution of phonomicrosurgical management. Laryngoscope 1995;105: 1–51.

12. Holliday MA, Bones VM, Malekzadeh S, et al. Low-cost modular phonosurgery training station: development and validation. Laryngoscope 2015;125(6):1409–13.

13. Dedmon MM, Paddle PM, Phillips J, et al. Development and validation of a high-fidelity porcine laryngeal surgical simulator. Otolaryngol Head Neck Surg 2015;2: 1–7.

14. Fleming J, Kapoor K, Sevdalis N, et al. Validation of an operating room immersive microlaryngoscopy simulator. Laryngoscope 2012;122(5):1099–103.

15. Nixon IJ, Palmer FL, Ganly I, et al. An integrated simulator for endolaryngeal surgery. Laryngoscope 2012;122(1):140–3.

16. Contag SP, Klein AM, Blount AC, et al. Validation of a laryngeal dissection module for phonomicrosurgical training. Laryngoscope 2009;119:211–5.

17. Cakmak H, Maass H, Kuhnapfel U. VS One, a virtual reality simulator for laparoscopic surgery. Minim Invasive Ther Allied Technol 2005;14(3):134–44.

18. Gallagher AG, Ritter EM, Champion H, et al. Virtual reality simulation for the operating room: proficiency-based training as a paradigm shift in surgical skills training. Ann Surg 2005;241:364–72.

19. Lioufas PA, Quayle MR, Leong JC, et al. 3D printed models of cleft palate pathology for surgical education. Plast Reconstr Surg Glob Open 2016;4(9):e1029.

20. Kavanagh KR, Cote V, Tsui Y, et al. Pediatric laryngeal simulator using 3D printed models: a novel technique. Laryngoscope 2017;127(4):E132–7.

21. Awad Z, Patel B, Hayden L, et al. Simulation in laryngology training; what should we invest in? Our experience with 64 porcine larynges and a literature review. Clin Otolaryngol 2015;40(3):269–73.

22. Zambricki EA, Bergeron JL, DiRenzo EE, et al. Phonomicrosurgery simulation: a low-cost teaching model using easily accessible materials. Laryngoscope 2016; 126(11):2528–33.

23. Zeitels SM, Franco RA, Dailey SH, et al. Office-based treatment of glottal dysplasia and papillomatosis with the 585-nm pulsed dye laser and local anesthesia. Ann Otol Rhinol Laryngol 2004;113(4):265–76.

24. Zeitels SM, Akst L, Burns JA, et al. Office based 532nm pulsed-KTP laser treatment of glottal papillomatosis and dysplasia. Ann Otol Rhinol Laryngol 2006;115: 679–85.
25. Zeitels SM, Akst L, Burns JA, et al. Pulsed angiolytic laser treatment of ectasias and varices in singers. Ann Otol Rhinol Laryngol 2006;115:571–80.
26. Broadhurst MS, Kobler JB, Burns JA, et al. Chick chorioallantoic membrane (CAM) as a model to simulate human true vocal folds. Ann Otol Rhinol Laryngol 2007;116(12):917–21.
27. Higbie E. The behavior of the virus of equine encephalomyelitis on the chorioallantoic membrane of the developing chick. J Bacteriol 1935;29:399–406.
28. Kimel S, Hammer-Wilson M, Gottfried V, et al. Demonstration of synergistic effects of hyperthermia and photodynamic therapy using the chick chorioallantoic membrane model. Lasers Surg Med 1992;12:432–40.
29. Ainsworth TA, Kobler JB, Loan GJ, et al. Simulation model for transcervical laryngeal injection providing real-time feedback. Ann Otol Rhinol Laryngol 2014; 123(12):881–6.
30. Cabrera-Muffly C, Clary MS, Abaza M. A low-cost transcervical laryngeal injection trainer. Laryngoscope 2016;126(4):901–5.
31. Amin M, Rosen CA, Simpson CB, et al. Hands-on training methods for vocal fold injection education. Ann Otol Rhinol Laryngol 2007;116(1):1–6.
32. Colt HG, Crawford SW, Galbraith O 3rd. Virtual reality bronchoscopy simulation: a revolution in procedural training. Chest 2001;120(4):1333–9.
33. Blum MG, Powers TW, Sundaresan S. Bronchoscopy simulator effectively prepares junior residents to competently perform basic clinical bronchoscopy. Ann Thorac Surg 2004;78(1):287–91.
34. Salud LH, Peniche AR, Salud JC, et al. Toward a simulation and assessment method for the practice of camera-guided rigid bronchoscopy. Stud Health Technol Inform 2011;163:535–41.
35. Deutsch ES, Dixit D, Curry J, et al. Management of aerodigestive tract foreign bodies: innovative teaching concepts. Ann Otol Rhinol Laryngol 2007;116(5): 319–23.
36. Deutsch ES. High-fidelity patient simulation mannequins to facilitate aerodigestive endoscopy training. Arch Otolaryngol Head Neck Surg 2008;134(6):625–9.
37. Deutschmann MW, Yunker WK, Cho JJ, et al. Use of a low-fidelity simulator to improve trans-nasal fiber-optic flexible laryngoscopy in the clinical setting: a randomized, single-blinded, prospective study. J Otolaryngol Head Neck Surg 2013; 42(1):35–9.
38. Laeeq K, Pandian V, Skinner M, et al. Learning curve for competency in flexible laryngoscopy. Laryngoscope 2010;120(10):1950–3.
39. De Oliveira GS Jr, Glassenberg R, Chang R, et al. Virtual airway simulation to improve dexterity among novices performing fiberoptic intubation. Anaesthesia 2013;68(10):1053–8.
40. Aho JM, Thiels CA, Al Jamal YN, et al. Every surgical resident should know how to perform a cricothyrotomy: an inexpensive cricothyrotomy task trainer for teaching and assessing surgical trainees. J Surg Educ 2015;72(4):658–61.
41. Wong DT, Prabhu AJ, Coloma M, et al. What is the minimum training required for successful cricothyroidotomy?: a study in mannequins. Anesthesiology 2003; 98(2):349–53.
42. Friedman Z, You-Ten KE, Bould MD, et al. Teaching lifesaving procedures: the impact of model fidelity on acquisition and transfer of cricothyrotomy skills to performance on cadavers. Anesth Analg 2008;107(5):1663–9.

43. Proctor MD, Campbell-Wynn L. Effectiveness, usability, and acceptability of haptic-enabled virtual reality and mannequin modality simulators for surgical cricothyroidotomy. Mil Med 2014;179(3):260-4.

44. Jayaraman V, Feeney JM, Brautigam RT, et al. The use of simulation procedural training to improve self-efficacy, knowledge, and skill to perform cricothyroidotomy. Am Surg 2014;80(4):377-81.

45. Gardiner Q, White PS, Carson D, et al. Technique training: endoscopic percutaneous tracheostomy. Br J Anaesth 1998;81(3):401-3.

Advanced Pediatric Airway Simulation

Charles M. Myer IV, MD[a],*, Noel Jabbour, MD, MS[b]

KEYWORDS

• Pediatric airway • Airway foreign body • Bronchoscopy • Simulation • Education

KEY POINTS

- Pediatric airway surgery is an ideal target for simulation given the limited case exposure, unique instrumentation, and shared airway.
- The use of a high-fidelity simulator for pediatric airway endoscopy scenarios allows for integration of procedural technical competency training with interdisciplinary crisis resource management.
- Limited simulation models exist for practice of more complex endoscopic airway procedures and open surgical techniques. Further development of validated simulators and integration of assessment tools will allow for improved surgical training.
- The use of simulation, including in situ sessions inside the operating room, is ideal for refining care delivery algorithms, especially in high-risk low-frequency events, such as pediatric aerodigestive foreign body ingestion.

INTRODUCTION

Pediatric airway cases often involve the shared management of the airway with anesthesia personnel, frequently without endotracheal intubation and using intermittent ventilation on airways undergoing surgical manipulation. Complex equipment must be assembled and handled by operating room (OR) nurses and surgical technicians. Achieving a successful outcome relies not only on the technical skill of the surgeon, but also on the interaction between this group of professionals through teamwork and effective communication.

There are several unique aspects of the care of the infant and pediatric airway that differ from adult airway management: the small size of airway, the significantly shorter

Disclosure Statement: The authors have nothing to disclose.
[a] Division of Pediatric Otolaryngology, Department of Otolaryngology–Head and Neck Surgery, Cincinnati Children's Hospital Medical Center, University of Cincinnati College of Medicine, 3333 Burnet Avenue, MLC 2018, Cincinnati, OH 45229-3026, USA; [b] Department of Otolaryngology, Children's Hospital of Pittsburgh of UPMC, University of Pittsburgh, 4401 Penn Avenue, Faculty Pavilion, 7th Floor, Pittsburgh, PA 15224, USA
* Corresponding author.
E-mail address: charlie.myer@cchmc.org

Otolaryngol Clin N Am 50 (2017) 923–931
http://dx.doi.org/10.1016/j.otc.2017.05.004
0030-6665/17/© 2017 Elsevier Inc. All rights reserved.

time of apnea that is tolerated by children given lower pulmonary reserve, and the types of airway pathology seen in infants and children. These features coalesce to create a high-stakes environment, and when coupled with the low-frequency of pediatric airway cases, these events are prime targets for surgical education using simulation. This can apply to residents in training and practicing otolaryngologists. Foreign body aspiration is one such case.

The Centers for Disease Control and Prevention categorizes foreign body aspiration under the umbrella of "suffocation." There has been an increase in the rate of death by suffocation between 2000 and 2009. It is the leading cause of death by unintentional injury in children younger than 1 year of age. In this age group, it increased from 526 to 907 deaths per year from 2000 to 2009. Suffocation deaths are less common in the 1- to-4-year-old range, with 151 deaths in 2000 and 125 deaths in 2009.[1]

Before the introduction of instrumentation for airway endoscopy and foreign body removal in the early 1900s, aspirations were commonly fatal. Now, largely because of these advances, such aspiration events are nearly universally survivable with proper care. Endoscopy for foreign body removal is a potentially life-saving procedure, but it is a complex, multistep procedure, with instrumentation that is used exclusively for this procedure, making skill acquisition and retention of acquired competency difficult.

Despite the frequency of these events, given the temporal and geographic distribution, the exposure to pediatric aerodigestive foreign body cases in otolaryngology residency is variable, and has been estimated at 1.3 cases per resident per year.[2] There is therefore a need to shift the learning outside of the OR for such cases. Over the past 10 years, simulation has played a significant role in the training of otolaryngology residents in these procedures.

But simulation for pediatric airway management is not a novel concept. Chevalier Jackson used rag dolls, such as his "Michelle the Choking Doll," to demonstrate his technique for foreign body removal and for emergency tracheostomy.[3] From foreign body removals to tracheostomy to complex airway reconstruction, simulated surgery of the pediatric airway can play a key role in the training of otolaryngologists for high-stakes, low-frequency airway emergencies and for more routine endoscopic and open airway procedures.

Recent advances in the quality of simulators and the ability to assess trainee performance broadens the application for simulation in otolaryngology surgical education. This article covers the use of simulation for pediatric aerodigestive foreign body management and other pediatric airway procedures. The final section covers recent technological advances in airway simulation and discusses the potential application of these advances for the future of pediatric airway simulation.

SIMULATION FOR AIRWAY ENDOSCOPY AND AERODIGESTIVE FOREIGN BODIES

Endoscopic and laparoscopic surgical techniques lend themselves to simulation because of the complex psychomotor tasks necessary to manipulate unique instrumentation. The primary goal of simulation, that of deliberate practice to achieve or maintain proficiency, is especially relevant in endoscopic management of an airway foreign body in a child (a true high-acuity, low-frequency event). A learner who is "primed" through prior exposure to the concepts, equipment, and surgical steps before being involved in a live patient encounter may be able to better function inside the OR and achieve greater educational gains. This concept of a pretrained novice is especially important in these cases, where there is less opportunity to allow for the more traditional surgical educational apprenticeship model of increasing responsibility.[4]

Deutsch and colleagues reintroduced the concept of simulated practicum in additional the traditional surgical education ideals of didactics and case exposure in 2007.[5] In this case report, a high-fidelity infant mannequin was used to perform bronchoscopy for airway foreign body removal in a simulated OR environment. Simulation sessions were used to develop resident's endoscopic procedural skills, instrument knowledge, management of complications, and communication and leadership abilities.

This concept, using high-fidelity mannequins in the simulation of airway endoscopy and intervention, was then expanded into a course including additional learning modalities; lecture, animal laboratory sessions, virtual reality bronchoscopy, and standardized patient interactions. Course attendees perceived value in each modality and self-reported improvement in cognitive and technical skill acquisition.[6]

Likewise, further courses primarily using high-fidelity mannequins in the teaching of pediatric airway laryngoscopy/bronchoscopy intervention or foreign body management have found similar positive outcomes on learner self-assessments.[4,7–9] Although the initial studies suffer from the potential for significant response bias, further publications examining learner outcomes with more objective measures have shown improvement following the educational intervention.[4,9] At this time, there are no reports examining either retention or translation of acquired skills and knowledge outside of the simulation environment to the OR, a task made more difficult by the infrequency of foreign body aspiration and the small number of trainees.

Airway Endoscopy Simulators

Several surgical simulation models have been described for laryngoscopy and bronchoscopy interventions, from low-fidelity physical models, high-fidelity mannequins, biologic tissue, and animal models, to virtual reality with or with haptic feedback.[10,11] Several described simulation models for laryngoscopy and bronchoscopy are repurposed or expanded commercially available simulators developed primarily for other purposes. Although the anatomic realism of the laryngeal and tracheobronchial structures may not be exact, there is enough similarity to enable adequate recognition of anatomic structures and response to surgical manipulation. Each simulator has its advantages and disadvantages, and selection should be based on the learning objectives identified for each simulation and the target audience for intervention, keeping in mind cost and availability. When using live animals or ex vivo tissue for training purposes, ethical and infectious control issues must also be considered.

Simulation Exercises

Although task trainers or animal models enable isolated procedural skill development, the use of high fidelity simulators allows incorporation of technical training into a robust clinical scenario. With the simulator's ability to alter its physiologic state, such as cardiac output, ventilation, and oxygenation, it can respond to learner manipulation with measurable responses. Additional personnel may be used to assist in caring for the "patient," including anesthesiologists, nurses, and ancillary personnel (**Fig. 1**). As compared to a static model, this enhances realism and allows for the incorporation of learning objectives outside of the technical mastery of a procedure, such as situational awareness, crisis resource management, and leadership skills. Thus, each simulation scenario can be further tailored to match the level of the trainee.

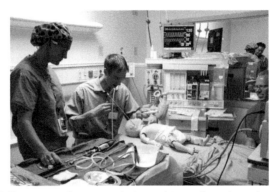

Fig. 1. A high-fidelity neonatal mannequin is used to perform bronchoscopy with foreign body removal as part of a multidisciplinary simulation scenario incorporating operating room personnel and anesthesia.

Examples showing the development of learning objectives and the use of simulation scripting in pediatric airway endoscopy simulation are found in the review by Cavel and colleagues.[12]

Skill Assessment

The development and adoption of Objective Structured Assessment Technical Skills (OSATS) enables further advances in simulator development and incorporation into otolaryngology education. By facilitating accurate assessment of trainee competence, deficiencies in the learner may be identified. Similarly, one may evaluate the efficacy of an education interventions or simulation to the acquisition of skills and the educational intervention can be identified. Through the routine use of these objective measures residency training, the ability of simulation training to translate from the simulation laboratory to the OR may be better determined. These tools are also useful adjuncts in guiding simulation debriefing. Several OSATS examining performance of airway endoscopy have been validated in either live patient encounters[13,14] or simulation models.[4,15]

In Situ Simulation

Simulations involving endoscopic airway evaluation and intervention can be exported from the simulation laboratory environment to an in-hospital, or in situ, environment. The benefits of performing simulation scenarios in the usual clinical environment include improved experiential learning and improved training efficiency. By incorporating simulation into the actual work environment in which the training is to be used, learners may achieve better translation of the gained knowledge.[16] Additionally, in situ simulation improves training efficiency by allowing easier access to personnel and may be more affordable than access to a simulation center.[16,17] Volk and colleagues[18] incorporated pediatric airway emergency simulations into the OR and intensive care unit environment for training otolaryngology residents, reporting the improved ability to complete simulation education because of the decreased impact on patient care and improved resident availability. However, the most important outcome of in situ simulation may be the identification of latent safety threats in the clinical environment and knowledge gaps in the delivery of multidisciplinary care, as noted in this and other studies of in situ simulation in pediatric facilities.[18–22]

SIMULATION FOR OPEN AIRWAY SURGERY

With the increasing acceptance and integration of simulation in otolaryngologic training, including temporal bone dissection, endoscopic sinus surgery, and the aforementioned airway endoscopy and bronchoscopy techniques, the use of simulation for acquisition of technical skills in other airway procedures has emerged. This enables trainees to gain proficiency and allows for competency assessment in anatomically complex procedures with minimal or no risk to patients. This concept is now supported in the most recent program requirements for otolaryngology by the Accreditation Council on Graduate Medical Education.[23]

Currently described models for advanced airway surgery focus primarily on endolaryngeal interventions, such as balloon dilation and phonomicrosurgery, or emergency airway management procedures, primarily cricothyroidotomy. These encompass task trainers of low- and high-fidelity, and ex vivo animal models and participation in animal laboratory sessions.[10,11] All of these models have limitations in availability, cost, or in the accurate representation of anatomy and translation of acquired skills. Many of the described microlaryngeal simulators are able to achieve training for similar procedures used in pediatric microlaryngology, such as supraglottoplasty or laryngeal cleft repair.

Simulation courses currently available offer animal laboratory experience to learn complex airway reconstruction techniques, often using porcine or canine models. Deutsch and colleagues[6] reported on the use of an animal laboratory session as part of a multimodality education event focusing on endoscopic airway skill development, finding high ratings for animal laboratory session in overall realism, manual realism, and development of psychomotor knowledge and skill when compared with high-fidelity mannequins and virtual reality. However, the cost, availability of suitable facilities, and ethical concerns limit the widespread adoption of animal laboratory sessions for routine education.

Despite the known limitations in using live animal laboratory sessions for surgical simulation, there is a lack of soft tissue anatomic models of the neck with realism in the areas of interest to the pediatric otolaryngologist or airway surgeon. A neck-dissection simulator that includes a laryngotracheal complex has been described; however, the utility of such a model in teaching airway surgery, such as tracheostomy, or more involved airway reconstruction is unknown.[24] Ianacone and colleagues[25] report favorably on the face validity and feasibility of an ex vivo ovine head and neck tissue model for use in simulation of tracheostomy, cricothyroidotomy, laryngofissure, medialization laryngoplasty, tracheal resection with slide tracheoplasty, laryngotracheoplasty, and laryngectomy. By using ex vivo tissue, which may be obtained from an abattoir, the expense, availability, and ethical concerns related to animal laboratory sessions are greatly reduced while maintaining the anatomic realism.

Patient-Specific Simulation

In comparison with the previously discussed generalizable models used for skill acquisition, the ability of rapid prototyping or additive manufacturing to model patient-specific anatomy allows for preoperative surgical planning and patient-specific surgical simulation, with the potential benefits of decreased operative time or complications.[26] Although common in craniofacial and oncologic reconstruction, it is not a commonly used technique for preoperative surgical planning in pediatric airway reconstruction to date.[27,28] Case reports have described the use of three-dimensional (3D) printing as an aid for anatomic evaluation of the airway and to assist in endoscopic stent placement and endotracheal intubation.[29–32]

FUTURE OF ADVANCED PEDIATRIC AIRWAY SIMULATION

Pediatric airway endoscopy simulation has changed significantly from the days of Chevalier Jackson's "Michelle the Choking Doll." These advances have involved improvements in the realism of the airway mannequins and task trainers, the environment of the simulation experience, and the ability to provide feedback on performance.

Although currently available simulators offer adequate realism in the supraglottic structures, there are few existing models with the exact anatomy of interest to pediatric otolaryngologists. That is, there are a myriad of upper airway simulators that are useful for intubation; this is largely because there are multiple specialties that would benefit from intubation training (emergency medicine, anesthesia, critical care, and first responders). The anatomy of the upper airway to the level of the larynx is acceptable in these models, but is lacking in the realism of the glottis, subglottis, trachea, and bronchial tree to the level necessary for more advanced otolaryngology procedures. There is a clear gap in the available airway simulators for more advanced pediatric airway surgery and a need for otolaryngologists to work with manufacturers of airway endoscopy simulators to develop models that may be used for realistic simulation of procedures involving the aerodigestive tract.

3D printing, sometimes referred to as additive manufacturing, has been a paradigm shift not only for clinical practice but also for simulation in otolaryngology. This technology most often involves development of a 3D model using computer-aided design, which is then printed layer by layer in two dimensions to create a final 3D structure. Several years ago, the cost of this technology was high, and it was only available in a small number of laboratories and academic centers. However, at the time of this writing, an entry-level 3D printer can be purchased for less than $300. This technology ushers in an era where it is possible to design and print patient-specific models for simulation and deliberate practice on a personal or institutional level.

In an excellent review on the subject, VanKoevering and colleagues[33] describe three potential uses for 3D printing in otolaryngology education: (1) patient education, (2) learner education, and (3) surgical simulation. Most of this work has been done in temporal bone and nasal/sinus anatomy. However, some reports have described its emerging role in pediatric airway simulation.

Jabbour and colleagues[9] reported the development of a model that had more realistic airway anatomy based on patient-specific airway anatomy from computed tomography and MRI scans. A 3D model was developed and a 3D-negative mold was then printed. This mold was used to make a silicone-based model that could be used for bronchoscopy simulation. The model had anatomy that was more realistic than latex-based commercially available models. However, the soft silicone was susceptible to easy tearing by novice users. This may add to the simulation realism but also affords limited model durability. In a similar fashion, Kavanagh and colleagues[34] described a method for printing pediatric laryngeal models for simulation that include such pathology as subglottic cysts, laryngomalacia, subglottic stenosis, or laryngeal cleft.

Advances in technology may also improve the opportunity for trainees to receive feedback and the type of assessment provided. Although currently existing OSATS can evaluate operative skills in pediatric airway endoscopy and foreign body removal with high interrater reliability,[4,13–15] they require the presence of an expert to observe the simulation. Because many pediatric airway procedures involve microscopes or endoscopes, video recording of the operative hands and the endoscopic view simultaneously can provide a means for assessment or for operative coaching, and potentially increasing the usefulness of independent practice.[35] The use of load/force sensors to provide objective measures, such as the pressure applied by the laryngoscope to the upper dentition or applied by the surgeon to the handle of the foreign body forceps, have also been described.[9] Sensors can similarly be placed throughout the airway to objectively measure forces that may result in injury in real-life scenarios.

In addition to procedural training, simulation involving the pediatric airway is used to improve patient safety and quality assurance. The use of simulation in selecting instrumentation for purchase by a hospital system has been described. Roberts and colleagues[36] used neonatal, child, and adult airway mannequins to assess the preference between two laryngoscope brands for purchase. A total of 34 health care providers used the laryngoscopes for simulated intubation. The authors advocate use of simulation to allow providers to compare products and declare preferences for medical equipment purchases.

Johnson and colleagues[19] described the use of in situ simulation to develop a patient care pathway for critical pediatric airway obstruction. Using 12 simulation scenarios of a 4 year old with witnessed grape aspiration, the authors compared the response of the health care team for six scenarios performed before implementation of a new patient care pathway and six scenarios performed after implementation of the pathway. The novel pathway, which involved the development of a critical airway team, algorithm, and paging system, resulted in decreased time for otolaryngology to arrive, from 7.8 minutes to 5.0 minutes, and decreased time until specialized airway equipment was available.

Taken together, these two studies demonstrate the use of simulation to evaluate the means by which equipment is purchased, stored, and made available when needed for critical situations. These techniques can be used to analyze the current method by which pediatric airway obstruction is managed in an institution. When seconds and minutes are critical to patient survival and outcomes, such simulation tested and optimized protocols are extremely valuable but currently underused.

SUMMARY

Although there is nearly a century of history in pediatric airway endoscopy simulation, it is only recently that currently available technology has been integrated to improve surgical simulation in all aspects of pediatric airway surgery. By incorporating advanced methods of surgical simulation into training programs, skill acquisition and clinical competency is improved while maintaining patient safety. With recent technological advances, the realm of possibilities for surgical simulation is rapidly expanding. Collaboration between surgeons and manufacturers will be necessary to create more realistic and accessible models.

REFERENCES

1. Gilchrist J, Ballesteros MF, Parker EM. Vital signs: unintentional injury deaths among persons aged 0–19 years — United States, 2000–2009. MMWR Morb Mortal Wkly Rep 2012;61(15):270–6.
2. Shah RK, Patel A, Lander L, et al. Management of foreign bodies obstructing the airway in children. Arch Otolaryngol Head Neck Surg 2010;136(4):373–9.
3. Jackson C. Chevalier Jackson demonstrating Michelle the choking doll. In: The College of Physicians of Philadelphia Digital Library. 2015. Available at: http://www.cppdigitallibrary.org/items/show/4415. Accessed December 27, 2016.
4. Griffin GR, Hoesli R, Thorne MC. Validity and efficacy of a pediatric airway foreign body training course in resident education. Ann Otol Rhinol Laryngol 2011; 120(10):635–40.

5. Deutsch ES, Dixit D, Curry J, et al. Management of aerodigestive tract foreign bodies: innovative teaching concepts. Ann Otol Rhinol Laryngol 2007;116(5): 319–23.

6. Deutsch ES, Christenson T, Curry J, et al. Multimodality education for airway endoscopy skill development. Ann Otol Rhinol Laryngol 2009;118(2):81–6.

7. Malekzadeh S, Malloy KM, Chu EE, et al. ORL emergencies boot camp: using simulation to onboard residents. Laryngoscope 2011;121:2114–21.

8. Gause CD, Hsiung G, Schwab B, et al. Advances in pediatric surgical education: a critical appraisal of two consecutive minimally invasive pediatric surgery training courses. J Laparoendosc Adv Surg Tech A 2016;26(8):663–70.

9. Jabbour N, Reihsen T, Sweet RM, et al. Psychomotor skills training in pediatric airway endoscopy simulation. Otolaryngol Head Neck Surg 2011;145(1):43–50.

10. Javia L, Deutsch ES. A systematic review of simulators in otolaryngology. Otolaryngol Head Neck Surg 2012;147(6):999–1011.

11. Musbahi O, Aydin A, Al Omran Y, et al. Current status of simulation in otolaryngology: a systematic review. J Surg Educ 2017;74(2):203–15.

12. Cavel O, Giguere C, Lapointe A, et al. Training: simulating pediatric airway. Pediatr Clin North Am 2013;60:993–1003.

13. Ishman SL, Brown DJ, Boss EF, et al. Development and pilot testing of an operative competency assessment tool for pediatric direct laryngoscopy and rigid bronchoscopy. Laryngoscope 2010;120:2294–300.

14. Ishman SL, Benke JR, Johnson KE, et al. Blinded evaluation of interrater reliability of an operative competency assessment tool for direct laryngoscopy and rigid bronchoscopy. Arch Otolaryngol Head Neck Surg 2012;138(10):916–22.

15. Jabbour N, Reihsen T, Payne NR, et al. Validated assessment tools for pediatric airway endoscopy simulation. Otolaryngol Head Neck Surg 2012;147(6):1131–5.

16. Patterson MD, Blike GT, Nadkarni VM. In situ simulation: challenges and results. In: Henriksen K, Battles JB, Keyes MA, et al, editors. Advances in patient safety: new directions and alternative approaches (vol. 3: performance and tools). Rockville (MD): Agency for Healthcare Research and Quality (US); 2008.

17. Fehr JJ, Honkanen A, Murray DJ. Simulation in pediatric anesthesiology. Paediatr Anaesth 2012;22:988–94.

18. Volk MS, Ward J, Irias N, et al. Using medical simulation to teach crisis resource management and decision-making skills to otolaryngology housestaff. Otolaryngol Head Neck Surg 2011;145(1):35–42.

19. Johnson K, Geis G, Oehler J, et al. Simulation to implement a novel system of care for pediatric critical airway obstruction. Arch Otolaryngol Head Neck Surg 2012;138(10):907–11.

20. Wheeler DS, Geis G, Mack EH, et al. High-reliability emergency response teams in the hospital: improving quality and safety using in situ simulation training. BMJ Qual Saf 2013;22(6):507–14.

21. Patterson MD, Geis GL, Falcone RA, et al. In situ simulation: detection of safety threats and teamwork training in a high risk emergency department. BMJ Qual Saf 2013;22(6):468–77.

22. Geis GL, Pio B, Pendergrass TL, et al. Simulation to assess the safety of new healthcare teams and new facilities. Simul Healthc 2011;6(3):125–33.

23. Accreditation Council for Graduate Medical Education. ACGME Program Requirements for Graduate Medical Education in Otolaryngology. 2016. Available at: https://www.acgme.org/Portals/.../ProgramRequirements/280_otolaryngology_2016.pdf. Accessed January 4, 2017.

24. Griffin GR, Rosenbaum S, Hecht S, et al. Development of a moderate fidelity neck-dissection simulator. Laryngoscope 2013;123:1682–5.
25. Ianacone DC, Gnadt BJ, Isaacson G. Ex vivo ovine model for head and neck surgical simulation. Am J Otolaryngol 2016;37:272–8.
26. Martelli N, Serrano C, van den Brink H, et al. Advantages and disadvantages of 3-dimensial printing in surgery: a systematic review. Surgery 2016;159:1485–500.
27. Chan HHL, Siewerdsen JH, Vescan A, et al. 3D rapid prototyping for otolaryngology – head and neck surgery: applications in image-guidance, surgical simulation and patient-specific modeling. PLoS One 2015;10(9):e0136370.
28. Kaye R, Goldstein T, Zeltsman D, et al. Three dimensional printing: a review on the utility within medicine and otolaryngology. Int J Pediatr Otorhinolaryngol 2016;89:145–8.
29. Han B, Liu Y, Zhang X, et al. Three-dimensional printing as an aid to airway evaluation after tracheostomy in a patient with laryngeal carcinoma. BMC Anesthesiol 2016;16:6.
30. Bustamante S, Bose S, Bishop P, et al. Novel application of rapid prototyping for simulation of bronchoscopic anatomy. J Cardiothorac Vasc Anesth 2014;28(4): 1122–5.
31. Miyazaki T, Yamasaki N, Tsuchiya T, et al. Airway stent insertion simulated with a three-dimensional printed airway model. Ann Thorac Surg 2015;99:e21–23.
32. Wilson CA, Arthurs OJ, Black AE, et al. Printed three-dimensional airway model assists planning of single-lung ventilation in a small child. Br J Anaesth 2015; 115(4):616–20.
33. VanKoevering KK, Hollister SJ, Green GE. Advances in 3-dimensional printing in otolaryngology: a review. JAMA Otolaryngol Head Neck Surg 2017;143:178.
34. Kavanagh KR, Cote V, Tsui Y, et al. Pediatric laryngeal simulator using 3D printed models: a novel technique. Laryngoscope 2016;127(4):E132–7. Available at: http://onlinelibrary.wiley.com/doi/10.1002/lary.26326/full. Accessed December 28, 2016.
35. Jabbour N, Sidman J. Assessing instrument handling and operative consequences simultaneously: a simple method for creating synced multicamera videos for endosurgical or microsurgical skills assessments. Simul Healthc 2011;6(5):299–303.
36. Roberts J, Sawyer T, Foubare D, et al. Simulation to assist in the selection process of new airway equipment in a children's hospital. Cureus 2015;7(9):e331.

Otologic Skills Training

Gregory J. Wiet, MBS, MD[a,b,c,*],
Mads Sølvsten Sørensen, MD, DMSc[d], Steven Arild Wuyts Andersen, MD, PhD[d,e]

KEYWORDS

- Surgical simulation • Otology training • Otology skills • Simulation training
- Surgical education

KEY POINTS

- Otology skills training ranges from simple procedures such as otoscopy to complex lateral skull base surgery, and simulation-based training of most otologic procedures is possible.
- Keys to effective learning of otologic skills in a simulation-based curriculum include distributed practice; deliberate practice; mastery learning; and directed, self-regulated learning with feedback.
- Future directions are likely to include further improvement of simulator fidelity and realism. However, the development of simulation-based curricula centered on adult learning theory, national efficacy studies, and validation of assessment strategies is required for learners to fully benefit from simulation technologies.

INTRODUCTION

Otologic skills training encompasses a range of procedures, including those that need to be mastered by all medical doctors, such as otoscopy; basic procedures needed by general otologists, such as myringotomy; and more advanced procedures, such as mastoidectomy and lateral skull base procedures. At present, in the United States, training in otologic skills in otolaryngology is accomplished throughout the 5-year course of clinical study. This training has traditionally consisted of a gradual increase in exposure and practice beginning with the most basic procedures, such as cerumen

Disclosures: G.J. Wiet has received research support from NIH/NIDCD 1R01-011321. M.S. Sørensen and S.A.W. Andersen have nothing to disclose and no conflicts of interest.
[a] Department of Otolaryngology, Nationwide Children's Hospital and The Ohio State University, 700 Children's Drive, Columbus, OH 43205, USA; [b] Department of Pediatrics, Nationwide Children's Hospital, 700 Children's Drive, Columbus, OH 43205, USA; [c] Department of Biomedical Informatics, The Ohio State University, 250 Lincoln Tower, 1800 Cannon Drive, Columbus, OH 43210, USA; [d] Department of Otorhinolaryngology–Head and Neck Surgery, Rigshospitalet, Blegdamsvej 9, Copenhagen DK-2100, Denmark; [e] Copenhagen Academy for Medical Education and Simulation, The Simulation Centre, Rigshospitalet, Blegdamsvej 9, Copenhagen DK-2100, Denmark
* Corresponding author. Department of Otolaryngology, Nationwide Children's Hospital, The Ohio State University, 700 Children's Drive, Columbus, OH.
E-mail address: gregory.wiet@nationwidechildrens.org

removal, and progressing to the more complex lateral skull base procedures. However, this time-honored training approach has come under pressure for change as a result of several factors, including less time available for individual teaching and an emphasis placed on patient safety whereby attending physicians are more sensitized to trainee involvement in patient care. Given these challenges that face all medical/surgical training programs, educators have increasingly looked toward simulation as a potential tool to mitigate these issues. In otolaryngology, several recent reviews of simulation activity noted that otology is one of the most developed with respect to simulation applications.[1,2] This article presents a summary of all otologic procedures in which simulation-based training is currently available and described in the literature, ranging from diagnostic procedures to mastoidectomy and more advanced procedures, including both physical and computer-based virtual-reality (VR) models. The article is divided based on procedure type, and, where applicable, it addresses the need for training, target trainees, available training systems, evidence for efficacy in training, and means for assessment of technical skill. Key features of effective simulation-based training in otology and future directions are presented.

OTOSCOPY

Otoscopy is the visual examination of the ear canal and the tympanic membrane and is used to diagnose a wide range of common ear canal and middle ear diseases, such as external otitis, acute and serous otitis media, and tympanic membrane perforation, in addition to identifying infrequent but important disorders such as cholesteatoma that need referral for surgery. Otoscopy is a common procedure and a key skill for all clinicians, including general practitioners and pediatricians. Otologists most often prefer otomicroscopy to allow magnification and simultaneous procedures such as removal of cerumen but much of the following discussion applies to otomicroscopy training as well.

Otoscopy skills can be taught on peers or patients because they cause little discomfort. However, otoscopy relies on the coordination of the instrument and the examiner's visual field, making it difficult to supervise in the training situation and to ensure that a systematic approach is learned unless a video otoscope is routinely used for training with feedback. In addition, adequate exposure to the full range of disorders can be difficult to achieve: often, training consists of practical training on the patients supplemented by textbook/atlas images of disorders. Optimally, training in otoscopy consists of repeated hands-on practice with feedback of otoscope and patient handling while also directing a systematic approach to the examination. There is a need for improvement in otoscopy skills training because general practitioners and medical students have shown comparable but mediocre otoscopy skills.[3]

A range of simulation-based training models for otoscopy have been reported: mannequin models for otoscopy and pneumatic otoscopy (Spectrum Nasco, Newmarket, Ontario, Canada; and Limbs and Things, Bristol, United Kingdom),[4] a Web-based platform with three-dimensional (3D) models of the ear displayed on a computer screen,[5,6] and more advanced models with a variety of situations that can also track the otoscope for annotation[7] and provide automated feedback.[8] An otoscopy simulator (OtoSim Inc, Toronto, Ontario, Canada) has been widely marketed and consists of the physical interface of an adult auricle and external canal with a small light-emitting diode (LED) screen that displays scaled images of normal and pathologic tympanic membranes. The instructor can control which image is displayed and point out disorders from a laptop computer connected to the interface. Recently, the system was upgraded to include pneumatic otoscopy capabilities. There is some evidence that simulation-based training can increase medical students' confidence in otoscopy[9] and the diagnostic accuracy of residents.[10]

For the assessment of otoscopy skills in a pediatric setting, a standardized checklist for otoscopy performance evaluation (SCOPE) has been developed.[11] There are currently no widely used or accepted instruments for the assessment of otoscopy skills in adults or in simulation-based training of otoscopy.

MYRINGOTOMY AND TYMPANOPLASTY

Myringotomy is the incision of the tympanic membrane to equilibrate pressure or drain fluid from the middle ear and is often accompanied by the insertion of a tympanostomy tube or grommet. Myringotomy is the most common surgical procedure in otology and one of the first skills learned by otorhinolaryngology (ORL) trainees. Tympanoplasty is the reconstruction of the tympanic membrane with and without ossicular chain reconstruction and is typically performed by a surgical otologist.

Physical models of the tympanic membrane are commonly used for initial training of myringotomy with tympanostomy tube insertion. Numerous models have been described ranging from do-it-yourself models based on readily available materials[12] to more complex physical models.[13,14] In addition, a VR simulation model for myringotomy and tube insertion with supporting haptic feedback has been developed.[15–18] Although global rating scales and task-based checklists have been developed and validated[12,19] to assess for myringotomy with tube insertion competency, evidence to support the efficacy of myringotomy simulation training is limited and high-quality studies examining the transfer of skills to improved patient outcomes are needed (the SimTube project is discussed later).

Tympanoplasty with/without ossicular chain reconstruction is frequently taught on cadavers, with the exception of the plastic Pettigrew temporal bone model, which can incorporate relevant disease processes[14]; nevertheless, reports on tympanoplasty training are scant and evidence for efficacy is lacking.

MASTOIDECTOMY

Mastoidectomy involves drilling of the temporal bone mastoid air cells with the purpose of treating infection or disorders such as cholesteatoma or to gain access to the middle ear, the cochlea, or the sinodural angle for lateral skull base procedures. Basic understanding and competency in mastoidectomy is expected of all otologists and is an important part of ORL residency training.

Temporal bone surgery requires precise motor skills to handle the otosurgical drill and suction irrigation under the magnification of the operating microscope. In addition, the temporal bone anatomy is complex with vital anatomic structures such as the facial nerve, the chorda tympani, the sigmoid sinus, the dura mater, the vestibular organ, and the ossicles. These complex skills are typically taught through cadaveric dissection during temporal bone courses or in training facilities with a temporal bone laboratory, all followed by supervised surgery. Cadaveric dissection was the gold-standard training modality for mastoidectomy even before evidence of its role in training recently began to emerge.[20,21] However, the availability of human temporal bones, in addition to the cost of maintaining facilities, among other issues considerably limits the availability of cadaveric dissection training for mastoidectomy. Plastic and plaster models,[14,22,23] and recently 3D printed temporal bones,[24,25] have been introduced to alleviate these issues; however, the physical properties and fidelity of vital structures in these models, along with costs, limit the adaptation of these simulators into mainstream temporal bone surgical training.

Several VR simulators have been developed and validated for temporal bone surgical training with the potential of immediate assessment of performance and monitoring of individual trainees' progress while providing automated feedback and tutoring. Most VR temporal bone simulators use a volumetric model that supports haptic interaction for drilling with force feedback and uses different technologies to accomplish 3D stereo graphics. VR simulators are based on either CT-derived data (Voxel-Man,[26] the Ohio State University,[27] the Stanford BioRobotics laboratory,[28] and the University of Melbourne[29]), or on cryosections of a fresh frozen human temporal bone (Visible Ear Simulator[30,31]).

Strong evidence exists to support the use of VR simulation training in temporal bone surgical skills training. First, novice versus expert performance can be discriminated in VR simulation of temporal bone surgery[32–34] and many simulator-based metrics correlate with experience.[1,35] Second, VR simulation performance has been shown to be similar to the dissection performance in trainees[36] and VR simulation training seems to be superior to training methods such as video demonstration.[37] Also, VR simulation training allows for self-directed training of mastoidectomy with an acceptable level of performance, minimizing the need for human instructional resources.[38] In addition, repeated VR simulation practice results in improved learning curves,[39,40] acceptable retention of the procedure skills,[41] and significantly increased cadaveric dissection performance.[42]

Several assessment tools for mastoidectomy performance and competency have been described for use in the operating room, cadaveric dissection laboratory or VR simulation setting. These tools incorporate global rating scales, task-based checklists, and/or final-product analysis. A recent review provides an excellent overview of the different mastoidectomy assessment tools and the current validity evidence for each tool.[43]

ADVANCED OTOLOGIC PROCEDURES

Surgical implantation of cochlear implants and other implantable hearing devices, as well as middle ear reconstruction using prostheses and stapes surgery, are considered advanced procedures of interest for subspecialist training in otology. At present, this advanced training is achieved on cadavers and supervised surgery because few training models are available beyond research prototypes. Physical models for the placement of stapes prosthesis include simulators using readily available materials,[44,45] the Pettigrew Temporal Bone Model with stapedotomy and prosthesis placement,[14] and models for electrode placement in cochlear implantation. In 2011, a prototype VR simulation model for cochlear implantation with haptic feedback was described.[46] To date, there is limited research on the training and assessment of advanced otologic skills; just a single report on the development and validation of an assessment tool for competency in cochlear implant surgery.[47]

KEY FEATURES OF EFFECTIVE SIMULATION-BASED OTOLOGIC SKILLS TRAINING
Repeated Practice and Mastery Learning

Studies have shown that 10 to 15 operative procedures are needed for technical and basic competency in mastoidectomy.[48,49] However, proficiency in surgical procedures requires substantially more practice (up to 100 procedures) but often at the cost of patient discomfort, longer procedural times, and increased risk of complications.[50] The learning curve must be considered and simulation-based training allows for repetitive practice tailored to the individual trainee's needs. Such mastery learning is crucial in competency-based education and marks a paradigm shift in surgical education, in which length of training or number of procedures had been the measured outcome. Mastery learning redefines the goals of training as consistent performance with an evidence-based level of proficiency.[51] To achieve mastery learning, deliberate practice with feedback is key.[52–54] The controlled environment of a simulation setting offers an ideal platform for setting standards and defining mastery levels before training on cadavers or supervised surgery. For otologic procedures, these standards have yet to be defined using validated assessment tools.

Practice Organization

Supported by established theory of motor skills learning and current evidence in other surgical procedures, a study of learning curves in VR simulation-based training of mastoidectomy found that practice should be distributed. Practice sessions should be short (3–4 procedures per session) and spaced (by at least 3 days) for optimal learning.[39] In reality, dissection training is often organized as short and intense courses; massed practice consistently leads to suboptimal skills acquisition, retention, and transfer.[41,55–57] The positive effect of distributed practice can be attributed to time-dependent consolidation of memory[57] and, even for a simple procedure such as myringotomy, spacing practice by a single day is insufficient in improving novice performance.[58] Therefore, the increasingly popular so-called ORL surgical boot camps[59,60] with simulation-based, massed practice of a range of surgical skills may have limited long-term effectiveness for learning otologic skills.

Instructional Design, Feedback, and Self-directed Training

The single most important feature of effective simulation-based training is feedback.[61] One of the benefits of VR simulation is the potential for self-directed learning using simulator-integrated tutoring, guidance, and feedback, eliminating the need for human instructors, who are often limited by clinical duties and other time constraints. A directed and self-regulated approach promotes independent learning in a structured setting with a strong instructional design.[62] In mastoidectomy, 2 hours of self-directed VR simulation training with automated guidance has been found to be superior to small-group tutorials using operative videos and temporal bone models[63] and, in a different study, was found to increase subsequent dissection performance by 52%.[42]

In self-directed training, repeated practice steeply increased the performance of novices, plateauing after 9 repetitions,[39] with intact retention after 3 months of non-practice.[41] Simulator-integrated tutoring in VR simulation training of mastoidectomy increases the slope of the initial part of the learning curve, further supporting directed, self-regulated learning.[39] Nevertheless, many novices have difficulty knowing when to stop drilling or may injure vital structures in the anatomic boundaries of the mastoidectomy, which may lead to a suboptimal performance.[64] These concerns for novices suggest that self-directed training in mastoidectomy could be further improved through instructional design with specific and explicit process goals.[65]

Evidence-Based Training

Although research in otologic skills training has focused on mastoidectomy, evidence from other technical skills and procedural training supports distributed and deliberate practice; mastery learning; and directed, self-regulated techniques in simulation-based training. A major challenge is the implementation of these evidence-based principles into high-quality training programs in otology. More importantly, simulation-based training should be "part of a coherent strategy based on clear educational aims and must mirror actual practice." [66] Furthermore, training should use scaffolding, in which subsequent learning experiences such as dissection training and supervised surgery build further on the skills acquired in simulation. Ultimately, this leads to improved patient outcomes.

FUTURE DIRECTIONS

Although there have been many technological advances leading to sophisticated computer-based simulators, the examples discussed earlier show several novel non–computer-based simulators. However, it needs to be recognized by those developing otologic simulators that the simulators are simply tools that need to be integrated into well-thought-out educational approaches using adult learning theory such as accurate needs assessments/task analysis, curriculum development, and valid outcome measures in addition to the key features for effective learning noted earlier. For those involved in the growing simulation movement, the challenge to not focus on the simulators but on the educational goals cannot be overemphasized. A well-designed simulator is one that meets an educational goal and not just a physical model or computer program that tries to replicate the real-life experience. The challenges that remain include development of universally agreed-on and valid measures of assessment, development of national and/or international frameworks for performing large-scale randomized controlled trials to provide robust statistical evidence for efficacy emphasizing patient outcomes as the ultimate measure of successful interventions. Learning effectiveness studies must move from more subjective types of evidence, such as self-assessments (Kirkpatrick level 1) to demonstration of results (Kirkpatrick level 4).[67] For these goals to be achieved, a firm commitment must be championed not only from grass-roots training programs but also from the health care education governance bodies.

One current attempt at instituting a nationwide otologic simulation skills training program that meets these criteria is underway. The SimTube project, sponsored by the American Academy of Otolaryngology Head and Neck Surgery Foundation, Inc, was developed by the Simulation Task Force to attempt to institute a large multicenter-based trial of a simulation-based training program for myringotomy and tube (M&T) insertion. The 3 hypotheses for this project include (1) a specialty-wide multi-institutional simulation study is feasible; (2) novices trained using the M&T simulator, compared with standard training, will achieve higher scores on both simulator and initial intraoperative objective structured assessment of technical skills (OSATS); and (3) novices trained on the simulator will reach competency sooner than those not trained on the simulator. The simulator used in this study was previously described by Malekzadeh and colleagues.[12] The protocol includes a randomized controlled trial of novice otolaryngology trainees randomized either to traditional training at their home institutions or traditional training plus initially supervised and then independent training using the simulator (**Fig. 1**). Study subjects are assessed using a validated assessment tool modified from the Malekzadeh and colleagues[12] study, which includes both a task-based checklist and global rating scale. Assessments are made on all subjects initially using the simulator after each has watched an online video, after 1 hour of training on the simulator for those randomized to simulator training, and then subsequently while the subject is performing the procedure on real patients. Assessments are continued until the rater judges the subject as competent. Study subjects keep records of how many procedures they perform until deemed competent as well as of the time spent using the simulator. At present, there are 65 out of the 106 otolaryngology training programs across the United States enrolled in the project, with the goal to recruit a total of 314 study subjects (157 per arm). This ongoing study

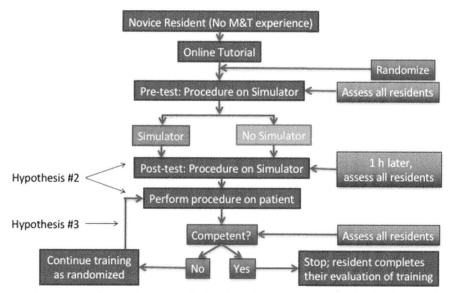

Fig. 1. The SimTube study protocol showing the nationwide randomized controlled simulation-based training project for myringotomy and tube placement. See text for information regarding the 3 hypotheses of the study. (*Courtesy of* the American Academy of Otolaryngology—Head and Neck Surgery Foundation, Alexandria, VA; with permission.)

is one of the first of its kind to be implemented in otolaryngology. Even if the study does not show a statistically significant difference between the 2 study arms, it will provide a framework and infrastructure to perform more definitive studies of simulation-based training programs.

Advancement in computer-based, VR systems deserves special mention when future directions are addressed. Despite these systems having been present for more than 10 years they have not reached mainstream training. There seem to be several limitations with these systems, including suboptimal realism, lack of scientifically rigorous validation studies, cost, and lack of valid and reliable assessment tools to assess performance after training.[68] The lack of realism has been pointed out in particular in temporal bone VR simulators. Although simulation training systems do not need to replicate reality, they do need to provide adequate fidelity to present key features of the real experience. In temporal bone surgery, one of the cornerstone skills that need to be developed is the identification of bone embedded landmark structures while drilling by thinning bone to a thickness that allows transillumination of the structure beneath, thus allowing identification of the structure before it is violated. To date, no system has achieved the ability to render bone in a virtual environment sufficiently to support practice of this skill. At present, visual rendering has progressed as a result of unique computer algorithms taking advantage of advancements in graphics processing units (**Figs. 2** and **3**).[69] Haptic rendering is another field of development, and development in this area continues.[70]

Furthermore, the lack of scientifically rigorous validation/outcome studies continues to limit integration of VR and other simulators into regular training programs.[1,68] Otolaryngology is not alone in this area because most studies of technology-enhanced simulation training and assessment in health professions have proved inadequate for modern psychometric research.[71] Most studies have weak designs

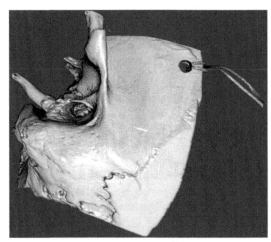

Fig. 2. Temporal bone rendered using a technique called global illumination. Global illumination is a graphics rendering technique that takes into account the distribution of light throughout a scene.

incorporating small numbers of study subjects and outmoded concepts of validity evidence.[72] The challenge is to develop and execute scientifically rigorous experiments comparing the effectiveness of these systems with standard training and organizing training programs in such a way as to leverage a large number of trainees at multiple institutions. This will require a national effort orchestrated by the larger organizations, such as the American Academy of Otolaryngology, the Otolaryngology Residency Review Committee, and The Society of University Otolaryngologists.

In addition, valid and reliable assessment of otologic skills is essential in a competency-based surgical curriculum, but providing useful feedback, opportunity to practice on a wide range of cases, and valid formative and summative assessment is resource intensive. VR simulation uniquely allows real-time feedback and automated assessment based on simulator registered metrics. In VR simulation training of mastoidectomy, for example, stroke and drilling technique can be used for effective and accurate feedback,[73] and simulator metrics can form the basis for automated assessment of the mastoidectomy performance.[74,75] With further refinement, and in combination with methodologies such as CUSUM (cumulative sum),[76,77] automated feedback and assessment provided by the simulator will in the future provide

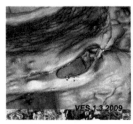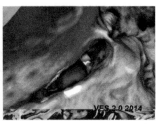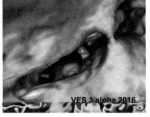

Fig. 3. Three examples from the Visible Ear Simulator 1 to 3 (VES 1–3) of a motif in which realistic transparency is crucial for navigation and safe drilling. In VES 3, natural transparency means that only the first few voxels below a bony surface are transparent. Internal luminescence and external vascular texture enhance the realism of the facial nerve as observed through a surgical microscope in its canal behind a thin layer of bone.

individualized, directed, self-regulated, and mastery learning in high-quality surgical training. There are currently several assessment tools that could potentially be integrated into VR systems for temporal bone surgery. A complete review of these is provided by Sethia and colleagues.[43]

Preoperative Planning

Although not directly thought of in relation to initial skills training, preoperative planning/practice is a type of just-in-time training and a review of otologic simulation platforms for presurgical planning was recently published.[78] The investigators found that there are several computer-based simulation platforms that have shown at least some form of feasibility for use in presurgical planning and practice. The systems reviewed use patient-specific image data that are then presented in 3D format within the simulator, allowing users to view and drill on the virtual temporal bone before the actual surgery. The key points were that the current systems were nascent for this application, that they have shown feasibility in that they can import patient-specific imaging studies in a timely fashion, but that they lack the fidelity to provide significant benefit for experienced surgeons. Perhaps with the integration of the fidelity enhancements noted earlier these systems will show efficacy in improving patient outcomes.

SUMMARY AND KEY POINTS

Simulation in otologic skills training is available across the spectrum, from otoscopy to advanced lateral skull base approaches involving the temporal bone. There exists a wide variation in educational approaches, validity evidence, and simulators. For educational programs to be effective, educators must integrate concepts of adult learning theory, such as distributed, self-regulated practice and mastery learning. Studies show the effectiveness of simulation training in otologic training through improved skills and performance. Otologic simulation continues to grow and future work will focus on improvements in simulator fidelity for advanced techniques and the development of universally accepted assessment tools for performance.

REFERENCES

1. Arora A, Hall A, Kotecha J, et al. Virtual reality simulation training in temporal bone surgery. Clin Otolaryngol 2015;40(2):153–9.
2. Deutsch ES, Wiet GJ, Seidman M, et al. Simulation activity in otolaryngology residencies. Otolaryngol Head Neck Surg 2015;153(2):193–201.
3. Fisher EW, Pfleiderer AG. Assessment of the otoscopic skills of general practitioners and medical students: is there room for improvement? Br J Gen Pract 1992;42(355):65–7.
4. Morris E, Kesser BW, Peirce-Cottler S, et al. Development and validation of a novel ear simulator to teach pneumatic otoscopy. Simul Healthc 2012;7(1):22–6.
5. Wickens B, Lewis J, Morris DP, et al. Face and content validity of a novel, web-based otoscopy simulator for medical education. J Otolaryngol Head Neck Surg 2015;44:7.
6. Stepniak C, Wickens B, Husein M, et al. Blinded randomized controlled study of a web-based otoscopy simulator in undergraduate medical education. Laryngoscope 2016;127(6):1306–11.
7. Davies J, Djelic L, Campisi P, et al. Otoscopy simulation training in a classroom setting: a novel approach to teaching otoscopy to medical students. Laryngoscope 2014;124(11):2594–7.

8. Magic V. EarSi Otoscope press release. Available at: https://www.vrmagic.com/simulators/news/article/new-otoscope-simulator/. Accessed October 18, 2016.

9. Lee DJ, Fu TS, Carrillo B, et al. Evaluation of an otoscopy simulator to teach otoscopy and normative anatomy to first year medical students. Laryngoscope 2015;125(9):2159–62.

10. Oyewumi M, Brandt MG, Carrillo B, et al. Objective evaluation of otoscopy skills among family and community medicine, pediatric, and otolaryngology residents. J Surg Educ 2016;73(1):129–35.

11. Paul CR, Keeley MG, Rebella G, et al. Standardized checklist for otoscopy performance evaluation: a validation study of a tool to assess pediatric otoscopy skills. MedEdPORTAL Publications 2016;12(10432):1–6.

12. Malekzadeh S, Hanna G, Wilson B, et al. A model for training and evaluation of myringotomy and tube placement skills. Laryngoscope 2011;121(7):1410–5.

13. Volsky PG, Hughley BB, Peirce SM, et al. Construct validity of a simulator for myringotomy with ventilation tube insertion. Otolaryngol Head Neck Surg 2009; 141(5):603–8.e1.

14. Pettigrew. Pettigrew temporal bones. Available at: http://www.temporal-bone.com/. Accessed November 2, 2016.

15. Sowerby LJ, Rehal G, Husein M, et al. Development and face validity testing of a three-dimensional myringotomy simulator with haptic feedback. J Otolaryngol Head Neck Surg 2010;39(2):122–9.

16. Wheeler B, Doyle PC, Chandarana S, et al. Interactive computer-based simulator for training in blade navigation and targeting in myringotomy. Comput Methods Programs Biomed 2010;98(2):130–9.

17. Ho AK, Alsaffar H, Doyle PC, et al. Virtual reality myringotomy simulation with real-time deformation: development and validity testing. Laryngoscope 2012;122(8): 1844–51.

18. Huang C, Cheng H, Bureau Y, et al. Face and content validity of a virtual-reality simulator for myringotomy with tube placement. J Otolaryngol Head Neck Surg 2015;44:40.

19. Schwartz J, Costescu A, Mascarella MA, et al. Objective assessment of myringotomy and tympanostomy tube insertion: a prospective single-blinded validation study. Laryngoscope 2016;126(9):2140–6.

20. Mowry SE, Hansen MR. Resident participation in cadaveric temporal bone dissection correlates with improved performance on a standardized skill assessment instrument. Otol Neurotol 2014;35(1):77–83.

21. Awad Z, Tornari C, Ahmed S, et al. Construct validity of cadaveric temporal bones for training and assessment in mastoidectomy. Laryngoscope 2015;125(10): 2376–81.

22. Awad Z, Ahmed S, Taghi AS, et al. Feasibility of a synthetic temporal bone for training in mastoidectomy: face, content, and concurrent validity. Otol Neurotol 2014;35(10):1813–8.

23. Vorwerk U, Begall K. Präparierübungen amvkünstlichen Felsenbein. HNO 1998; 46:246–51.

24. Hochman JB, Kraut J, Kazmerik K, et al. Generation of a 3D printed temporal bone model with internal fidelity and validation of the mechanical construct. Otolaryngol Head Neck Surg 2014;150(3):448–54.

25. Rose AS, Kimbell JS, Webster CE, et al. Multi-material 3D models for temporal bone surgical simulation. Ann Otol Rhinol Laryngol 2015;124(7):528–36.

26. Pflesser B, Petersik A, Tiede U, et al. Volume cutting for virtual petrous bone surgery. Comput Aided Surg 2002;7(2):74–83.

27. Wiet GJ, Stredney D, Sessanna D, et al. Virtual temporal bone dissection: an interactive surgical simulator. Otolaryngol Head Neck Surg 2002;127(1):79–83.

28. Morris D, Sewell C, Barbagli F, et al. Visuohaptic simulation of bone surgery for training and evaluation. IEEE Comput Graph Appl 2006;26(6):48–57.

29. O'Leary SJ, Hutchins MA, Stevenson DR, et al. Validation of a networked virtual reality simulation of temporal bone surgery. Laryngoscope 2008;118(6):1040–6.

30. Sorensen MS, Mosegaard J, Trier P. The visible ear simulator: a public PC application for GPU-accelerated haptic 3D simulation of ear surgery based on the visible ear data. Otol Neurotol 2009;30(4):484–7.

31. Sørensen MS, Dobrzeniecki AB, Larsen P, et al. The visible ear: a digital image library of the temporal bone. ORL J Otorhinolaryngol Relat Spec 2002;64(6): 378–81.

32. Khemani S, Arora A, Singh A, et al. Objective skills assessment and construct validation of a virtual reality temporal bone simulator. Otol Neurotol 2012;33(7): 1225–31.

33. Zirkle M, Roberson DW, Leuwer R, et al. Using a virtual reality temporal bone simulator to assess otolaryngology trainees. Laryngoscope 2007;117(2):258–63.

34. Sewell C, Morris D, Blevins N, et al. Achieving proper exposure in surgical simulation. Stud Health Technol Inform 2006;119:497–502.

35. Sewell C, Morris D, Blevins NH, et al. Validating metrics for a mastoidectomy simulator. Stud Health Technol Inform 2007;125:421–6.

36. Wiet GJ, Stredney D, Kerwin T, et al. Virtual temporal bone dissection system: OSU virtual temporal bone system: development and testing. Laryngoscope 2012;122(Suppl 1):S1–12.

37. Zhao YC, Kennedy G, Yukawa K, et al. Can virtual reality simulator be used as a training aid to improve cadaver temporal bone dissection? Results of a randomized blinded control trial. Laryngoscope 2011;121(4):831–7.

38. Zhao YC, Kennedy G, Hall R, et al. Differentiating levels of surgical experience on a virtual reality temporal bone simulator. Otolaryngol Head Neck Surg 2010;143(5 Suppl 3):S30–5.

39. Andersen SA, Konge L, Caye-Thomasen P, et al. Learning curves of virtual mastoidectomy in distributed and massed practice. JAMA Otolaryngol Head Neck Surg 2015;141(10):913–8.

40. Nash R, Sykes R, Majithia A, et al. Objective assessment of learning curves for the Voxel-Man TempoSurg temporal bone surgery computer simulator. J Laryngol Otol 2012;126(7):663–9.

41. Andersen SA, Konge L, Caye-Thomasen P, et al. Retention of mastoidectomy skills after virtual reality simulation training. JAMA Otolaryngol Head Neck Surg 2016;142(7):635–40.

42. Andersen SA, Foghsgaard S, Konge L, et al. The effect of self-directed virtual reality simulation on dissection training performance in mastoidectomy. Laryngoscope 2016;126(8):1883–8.

43. Sethia R, Kerwin TF, Wiet GJ. Performance assessment for mastoidectomy: state of the art review. Otolaryngol Head Neck Surg 2017;156(1):61–9.

44. Owa AO, Gbejuade HO, Giddings C. A middle-ear simulator for practicing prosthesis placement for otosclerosis surgery using ward-based materials. J Laryngol Otol 2003;117(6):490–2.

45. Mathews SB, Hetzler DG, Hilsinger RL Jr. Incus and stapes footplate simulator. Laryngoscope 1997;107(12 Pt 1):1614–6.

46. Todd CA, Naghdy F. Real-time haptic modeling and simulation for prosthetic insertion. World Acad Sci Eng Technol Proc 2011;(73):343–51.

47. Piromchai P, Kasemsiri P, Wijewickrema S, et al. The construct validity and reliability of an assessment tool for competency in cochlear implant surgery. Biomed Res Int 2014;2014:192741.

48. Francis HW, Masood H, Laeeq K, et al. Defining milestones toward competency in mastoidectomy using a skills assessment paradigm. Laryngoscope 2010; 120(7):1417–21.

49. Carr MM. Program directors' opinions about surgical competency in otolaryngology residents. Laryngoscope 2005;115(7):1208–11.

50. Eversbusch A, Grantcharov TP. Learning curves and impact of psychomotor training on performance in simulated colonoscopy: a randomized trial using a virtual reality endoscopy trainer. Surg Endosc 2004;18(10):1514–8.

51. Yudkowsky R, Park YS, Lineberry M, et al. Setting mastery learning standards. Acad Med 2015;90(11):1495–500.

52. Ericsson KA. Deliberate practice and the acquisition and maintenance of expert performance in medicine and related domains. Acad Med 2004;79(10 Suppl): S70–81.

53. Malik MU, Varela DA, Park E, et al. Determinants of resident competence in mastoidectomy: role of interest and deliberate practice. Laryngoscope 2013;123(12): 3162–7.

54. Bhatti NI, Ahmed A. Improving skills development in residency using a deliberate-practice and learner-centered model. Laryngoscope 2015;125(Suppl 8):S1–14.

55. Moulton CA, Dubrowski A, Macrae H, et al. Teaching surgical skills: what kind of practice makes perfect?: a randomized, controlled trial. Ann Surg 2006;244(3): 400–9.

56. Mackay S, Morgan P, Datta V, et al. Practice distribution in procedural skills training: a randomized controlled trial. Surg Endosc 2002;16(6):957–61.

57. Shea CH, Lai Q, Black C, et al. Spacing practice sessions across days benefits the learning of motor skills. Hum Movement Sci 2000;19(5):737–60.

58. Kesser BW, Hallman M, Murphy L, et al. Interval vs massed training: how best do we teach surgery? Otolaryngol Head Neck Surg 2014;150(1):61–7.

59. Malekzadeh S, Malloy KM, Chu EE, et al. ORL emergencies boot camp: using simulation to onboard residents. Laryngoscope 2011;121(10):2114–21.

60. Chin CJ, Chin CA, Roth K, et al. Simulation-based otolaryngology - head and neck surgery boot camp: 'how I do it'. J Laryngol Otol 2016;130(3):284–90.

61. Cook DA, Hamstra SJ, Brydges R, et al. Comparative effectiveness of instructional design features in simulation-based education: systematic review and meta-analysis. Med Teach 2013;35(1):e867–98.

62. Brydges R, Nair P, Ma I, et al. Directed self-regulated learning versus instructor-regulated learning in simulation training. Med Educ 2012;46(7):648–56.

63. Zhao YC, Kennedy G, Yukawa K, et al. Improving temporal bone dissection using self-directed virtual reality simulation: results of a randomized blinded control trial. Otolaryngol Head Neck Surg 2011;144(3):357–64.

64. Andersen SA, Konge L, Mikkelsen PT, et al. Mapping the plateau of novices in virtual reality simulation training of mastoidectomy. Laryngoscope 2016;127(4): 907–14.

65. Brydges R, Carnahan H, Safir O, et al. How effective is self-guided learning of clinical technical skills? It's all about process. Med Educ 2009;43(6):507–15.

66. Kneebone RL, Nestel D, Vincent C, et al. Complexity, risk and simulation in learning procedural skills. Med Educ 2007;41(8):808–14.

67. Kirkpatrick DL, Kirkpatrick JD, ebrary Inc. Implementing the four levels: a practical guide for effective evaluation of training programs. 1st edition. San Francisco (CA): Berrett-Koehler Publishers; 2007. Available at: http://site.ebrary.com/lib/yale/Doc?id=10205948.
68. Musbahi O, Aydin A, Al Omran Y, et al. Current status of simulation in otolaryngology: a systematic review. J Surg Educ 2016;74(2):203–15.
69. Zheng L, Chaudhari AJ, Badawi RD, et al. Using global illumination in volume visualization of rheumatoid arthritis CT Data. IEEE Comput Graph Appl 2014; 34(6):16–23.
70. Ghasemloonia A, Baxandall S, Zareinia K, et al. Evaluation of haptic interfaces for simulation of drill vibration in virtual temporal bone surgery. Comput Biol Med 2016;78:9–17.
71. Cook DA, Brydges R, Zendejas B, et al. Technology-enhanced simulation to assess health professionals: a systematic review of validity evidence, research methods, and reporting quality. Acad Med 2013;88(6):872–83.
72. Cook DA, Zendejas B, Hamstra SJ, et al. What counts as validity evidence? Examples and prevalence in a systematic review of simulation-based assessment. Adv Health Sci Educ 2014;19(2):233–50.
73. Wijewickrema S, Piromchai P, Zhou Y, et al. Developing effective automated feedback in temporal bone surgery simulation. Otolaryngol Head Neck Surg 2015; 152(6):1082–8.
74. Wiet G, Hittle B, Kerwin T, et al. Translating surgical metrics into automated assessments. Stud Health Technol Inform 2012;173:543–8.
75. Kerwin T, Wiet G, Stredney D, et al. Automatic scoring of virtual mastoidectomies using expert examples. Int J Comput Assist Radiol Surg 2012;7(1):1–11.
76. Bolsin S, Colson M. The use of the Cusum technique in the assessment of trainee competence in new procedures. Int J Qual Health Care 2000;12(5):433–8.
77. Biau DJ, Williams SM, Schlup MM, et al. Quantitative and individualized assessment of the learning curve using LC-CUSUM. Br J Surg 2008;95(7):925–9.
78. Sethia R, Wiet GJ. Preoperative preparation for otologic surgery: temporal bone simulation. Curr Opin Otolaryngol Head Neck Surg 2015;23(5):355–9.

Emerging Role of Three-Dimensional Printing in Simulation in Otolaryngology

Kyle K. VanKoevering, MD[a], Kelly Michele Malloy, MD[b],*

KEYWORDS

- Otolaryngology • Simulation • 3D printing • Stimulator • Surgical education
- Task trainers

KEY POINTS

- There are multiple three-dimensional (3D) printing technologies available. Understanding the basic principles and limitations of each can help determine the best manufacturing method for a simulator.
- Otologic simulators have been widely explored because of high anatomic complexity and limitations in cadaveric bones. Recent multimaterial models show promise in validation but are potentially costly.
- Sinonasal and laryngeal simulators are more recently being described with variable applications in endoscopic skill development.
- At a higher level, case-specific 3D simulations of high anatomic complexity have been described for surgical rehearsal before patient operations. Early reports have shown that surgical teams highly value the simulated experience.
- 3D printing has started to markedly affect simulation. As costs decline and the technology expands, applications in simulation will grow rapidly.

INTRODUCTION

In the era of personalized medicine, three-dimensional (3D) printing technology offers a mechanism for personalized surgical education as well. 3D printing can be used to create novel, complex simulators and task trainers that target specific anatomy and/or

Disclosures: The authors have no financial relationships or commercial interests to disclose.
[a] Department of Otolaryngology–Head and Neck Surgery, The Ohio State University Wexner Medical Center, 4000 Eye and Ear Institute, 915 Olentangy River Road, Columbus, OH 43212, USA; [b] Division of Head and Neck Oncology, Department of Otolaryngology–Head and Neck Surgery, Michigan Medicine, University of Michigan, 1904 Taubman Center, 1500 East Medical Center Drive, SPC 5312, Ann Arbor, MI 48109-5312, USA
* Corresponding author.
E-mail address: kellymal@med.umich.edu

Otolaryngol Clin N Am 50 (2017) 947–958
http://dx.doi.org/10.1016/j.otc.2017.05.006
0030-6665/17/© 2017 Elsevier Inc. All rights reserved.

surgical tasks; as such, once an educational gap is identified, 3D printing can be used to manufacture a model that is specific to the educational need and that can be produced rapidly.

Although most 3D printed simulators in otolaryngology are designed for surgical task training, some are translating to the bedside as models with which to practice for actual patient surgical care. The possibilities of 3D printing technology for surgical simulation and education are rapidly becoming realities, generating great excitement among surgeon educators in otolaryngology and related fields.

HISTORY AND BACKGROUND

3D printing has been introduced into medicine over the last decade with reports of lifesaving 3D printed airway splints,[1] bionic ears,[2] complex presurgical models for craniofacial reconstruction,[3] and a variety of other novel applications of the technology. 3D printing is creating new avenues in personalized medicine. It allows rapid manufacturing of highly customized devices that can be tailored to a patient's specific anatomy.

3D printing traces its roots back to the 1980s when it was described by Charles Hull for the aerospace and automotive industries.[4] The technology was initially developed to quickly prototype design ideas with inexpensive materials (hence the alternative name, rapid prototyping). Material development has expanded rapidly over recent years, allowing 3D printing in a complex array of colors, material density and stiffness to mimic organic tissue.[5] With expanded material capabilities, high-fidelity simulators can be created from anatomic cross-sectional imaging.

TECHNICAL ASPECTS OF THREE-DIMENSIONAL PRINTING

Functionally, 3D printing can be broken down into 5 basic steps[6]:

- First, a 3D object is virtually designed in a computer-aided design (CAD) modeling program. Anatomic 3D models can be created through a variety of modeling software using cross-sectional imaging in a process called segmentation.
- Next, the 3D object to be printed is virtually sliced into a stack of thin, two-dimensional (2D) slices. Slice thickness is based on the resolution of the printer and desired speed of print. Slice thickness can range from 5 to 500 μm.
- Third, a roadmap of each 2D slice is coded and transferred to the 3D printer.
- Fourth, the 3D printer prints the thin base slice on a platform. Once the first 2D slice is printed, the platform descends the defined slice thickness, and the next slice is printed. The process is repeated as each 2D slice is slowly stacked on the prior layers until the object is completed.
- Fifth, postprocessing is performed in which the object may be polished and support material (which can support overhangs as they are printed) is removed until the final product is created.

SEGMENTATION

In medical applications (including simulation), most 3D models are initially designed from patient-specific cross-sectional imaging data. DICOM images from computed tomography (CT) or MRI are typically uploaded into a segmentation program. The desired anatomy to be modeled is then selected in the program on a slice-by-slice basis through a variety of automated and manual process, segmenting the DICOM data into various elements (**Fig. 1**A, B). Using the DICOM image slice thickness (or CT/MRI resolution), the selected pixels of each 2D slice are stacked and blended into a 3D

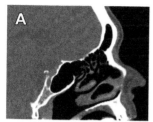
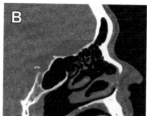
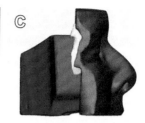

Fig. 1. Multipart nasal simulator. (*A*) Sagittal paramedian maxillofacial CT scan. (*B*) Representative segmentation of skin (*purple*), maxillary and frontal bone (*yellow*), and internal nasal anatomy (*pink*). (*C*) Virtual 3D model created from segmenting the skin/soft tissue (*purple*), facial skeleton (*yellow*), and internal nasal anatomy (*pink*).

model of the specified anatomy. Different components of the anatomy can then be joined into complex 3D objects for high-fidelity models (see **Fig. 1**C).

THREE-DIMENSIONAL PRINTING TECHNOLOGIES

Since its initial inception in the 1980s, several different printing technologies have been developed. In developing simulators, understanding the material properties, cost, and limitations of each printing technology can greatly influence the fidelity of the model. Some of the most common types of 3D printing technologies are reviewed here.

Stereolithography Printing

Stereolithography (SLA) printing is the technique initially described by Hull. The build platform is lowered into a liquid photopolymer, in which an ultraviolet (UV) laser light traces the pathway of the designated 2D slice, curing the liquid polymer into a solid. The platform descends the defined slice thickness until the hardened model is covered by a new layer of liquid polymer, and the process is repeated. This technology is capable of high resolution, smooth surface finish, and flexible prints, but offers limited color options (typically single-color prints) at fairly low costs.[7]

Fused Deposition Modeling

Fused deposition modeling (FDM) has become the most widely used printing technology in the consumer market. FDM uses a filament of thermoplastic polymer that is fed through a heated nozzle. The temperature must be beyond the glass transition temperature of the filament. The molten plastic is then finely extruded through the filament, where it rapidly cools and hardens in preparation for the next layer. This technology is readily available in consumer and commercial markets with a wide variety of thermoplastic properties, including some flexible materials. Limited multicolor prints are possible with multinozzle print heads.[8] Resolution and surface finish are typically modest, often requiring postprocessing. However, material and print costs are very low compared with other technologies.

Selective Laser Sintering

Selective laser sintering (SLS) uses finely pulverized (powdered) polymer that is uniformly spread across a print platform. Typically, a CO_2 laser then passes across the platform, sintering or binding the granules of raw material together. A variety of biocompatible polymers have been adapted to this printing technology, including high-strength materials and metal alloys. Initial setup costs are typically high because the machines are expensive and typically can print in a single color based on the material.[9,10] There are generally no requirements for support structures because the prints are suspended in a bed of unsintered powder; however, surface finish remains coarse given the granular starting material.

Inkjet Printing

Inkjet printing, similar to SLS, uses a powdered base material spread repeatedly across the build platform. A print head then deposits a binding resin in a process that mimics traditional 2D inkjet printers. The binding resin solidifies the powdered substrate where applied. The print head can often generate a wide array of complex color options for high-fidelity color prints without the need for support material, but maintains a granular surface finish with limited material properties.[10] This same approach has been used for so-called organic prints (bioplotting) in which a cellular suspension or various growth factors can be incorporated into the binding resin.

PolyJet Technology

PolyJet technology is one of the newest and most versatile print processes. It combines concepts of inkjet printing and SLA printing. The print head deposits liquid photopolymer across the build tray, which is subsequently cured by UV light. The liquid material allows for high-resolution, smooth finishes, whereas the multinozzle print heads allow for multicolor and multimaterial prints with high color complexity and variable mechanical properties.[7] However, these printers and materials are typically expensive, often available only in commercial environments, and do not have many biocompatible print options.

Silicone Molding

Silicone molding is now routinely being coupled with 3D printing. He and colleagues[11] describe the use of 3D modeling of complex anatomy, then creating a digital negative in the form of a mold. The molds can be 3D printed and then filled with silicone for realistic soft tissues. By way of example, **Fig. 2** shows an FDM-printed orbital anatomy (see **Fig. 2**A) with overlying silicone-molded facial soft tissues (see **Fig. 2**B). The silicone facial anatomy was created using 3D molds printed on the same FDM printer. The model can be used to simulate an orbital hematoma (see **Fig. 2**C).

CURRENT APPLICATIONS OF THREE-DIMENSIONAL PRINTING IN OTOLARYNGOLOGY

3D printing technology enables surgical educators to create anatomically accurate, complex models of head and neck anatomy for the purpose of surgical education. Models may be used for anatomic instruction or for procedural training. Some 3D printed simulators have even been developed to assist with surgical planning for patients. As this technology continues to be implemented across the subspecialties of

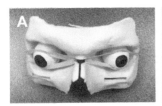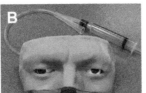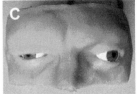

Fig. 2. 3D printed orbital simulator. (*A*) 3D printed facial skeleton with globes held in position with rubber bands. (*B*) Overlaid silicone face mask, molded in 3D printed molds. (*C*) Inflated Foley catheter in the posterior orbit can simulate proptosis.

otolaryngology there will be opportunities to measure its effect on surgical training and potentially on patient outcomes; to date, the current literature is limited to proof-of-concept or early validation studies. Unlike in virtual reality simulation, 3D printed models allow use of the actual surgical instruments, from forceps and suture to endoscopes and microscopes, during the surgical training. This enhances the reality, or fidelity, of the procedural simulations, irrespective of the materials used to print these models.

TEMPORAL BONE SIMULATORS

Perhaps the most widely described otolaryngologic 3D printed simulator in otolaryngology has been the temporal bone. The highly complex 3D anatomic relationships of the human temporal bone, as well as surgical approaches primarily focusing around bony removal, make the temporal bone an ideal candidate for high-fidelity simulation. Initial 3D printed temporal bones in the early 2000s focused on accurate representation of bony anatomy, often limited to single-material or dual-material models, generated from high-resolution CT scan. Suzuki and colleagues[12] published one of the first reports in 2004 using SLS printing to represent the bony anatomy with acceptable results, although limitations were seen in overall fidelity and retained support powder.

Since that early publication many other groups have described a wide array of temporal bone simulators on a variety of printing techniques. These techniques include SLA[13] and FDM,[14,15] which were largely limited to single material prints, although cavities could be filled with colored materials to simulate realism. These techniques scored modestly for realism with drilling experience. Inkjet prints provided added detail with incorporated color and realistic bony drilling.[16–18] The greatest limitation to the models was the frequent trapping of powdered substrate, which was a reflection of the complexity of the negative spaces of the middle ear and mastoid air cells. Hochman and colleagues[16] performed detailed mechanical testing to validate the most realistic inkjet printing resin compared with bone.

PolyJet prints have added further fidelity to the temporal bone prints. With a wide array of colors and material properties, this printing technology has shown promise in simulation. Rose and colleagues[19] describe their use of this technology and validation with otolaryngology residents and attendings, and scored better than average in all domains. Eight otolaryngology attendings completed validation reviews on the 3D printed models developed from a high-resolution clinical CT scan using a 10-question survey based on a 5-point Likert scale. The data were promising, and the investigators subsequently proceeded to a cadaveric temporal bone that underwent micro-CT for higher resolution modeling. The drilling and surveys were then repeated with 13 experienced otolaryngology residents and attendings. The average rating for the initial model was 4.2 out of 5 on the Likert scale compared with cadaveric temporal bone drilling, whereas the second model scored slightly higher in most domains, with an overall score of 4.3 out of 5. The investigators do not comment on the cost of each model, but conclude that the 3D models have potential value in otologic training.

OTHER OTOLOGIC SIMULATORS

In addition, 3D printing has been used to create models for other otologic procedures. Similar to temporal bone simulation, these other ear surgery simulators may promote surgical training in procedures that are less common; take a long time in practice to master; have a low tolerance for small errors; or use new technology, such as endoscopes.

CONGENITAL AURAL ATRESIA

Andrews and colleagues[20] reported on an early otologic application of 3D modeling in 1994, printing a plastic model of congenital aural atresia that could be drilled for surgical practice. Their proof-of-concept article reflects the early challenges of applying 3D printing to surgical simulation, including materials issues, negative space challenges (ie, how to remove negative material from cavities like the middle ear), and the limitations of thicker-sliced, less-refined CT scans.

ENDOSCOPIC EAR SURGERY

Simulation seems uniquely suited to training novices and experienced surgeons alike in new technologies. Barber and colleagues[21] identified a need for simulation for the new procedure of transcanal endoscopic ear surgery (TEES) in children. This procedure is different from binocular microscopic surgery of the ear, and surgeons need to master new technical skills in which they operate an endoscope in one hand and instruments in the other. Rather than using a single CT scan to print their models, they used normative data from anthropometric studies of the external auditory canal, and constructed a middle ear dome workspace where the endoscopic tasks would be performed (moving donuts from peg to peg within the middle ear dome). Printed in composite materials, the investigators argue that this produces a durable multiuse simulator that allows TEES practice. Barber and colleagues[21] do not report expert validation data, nor do they report the cost specific to their simulator production, only stating that this is a less expensive option than cadavers. They did report a short series of time trials of 6 trainees who used the simulator, noting that they improved their times with practice and with higher training levels.

AURICULAR RECONSTRUCTION

Auricular reconstruction undertaken with rib cartilage grafts is a technically challenging surgery with little room for error. Trainees and surgeons alike have identified a need to practice carving skills, both in general and for patient-specific cases. Berens and colleagues[22] describe using 3D printing to model pediatric rib and adjacent cartilage from a high-resolution CT chest scan of an 8-year-old boy. Using the negative model of the 3D reconstruction from the CT scan, they 3D printed a reusable mold in polylactic acid.

The investigators allowed for several types of material to be used to create rib cartilage graft simulators and compared them. Three expert microtia surgeons carved and sutured the grafts just as they would in surgery, rating the fidelity of the materials in multiple domains (**Fig. 3**): texture, firmness, carving, suturing, bending, and geometry. Higher starch/silicone ratio (2:1) models rated better than lower ratio preparations and vinyl polysiloxane, a material commonly used for dental impressions. Starch/silicone models were also most cost-effective, and fairly inexpensive at US$0.60 per trainer. The study did not report the cost of the 3D printer, technical expertise costs, or the cost of 3D printed mold.

Further validation studies are still needed for the higher ratio starch/silicone model. This model has exciting implications for resident and fellow training and maintains patient safety, as well as for experienced surgeons to practice carving before surgery. Future possibilities for patient-specific surgical rehearsal include using 3D printed models of an individual's own costal cartilage.

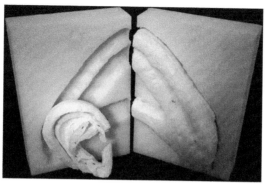

Fig. 3. Rib cartilage simulator designed from a silicone mixture in a 3D printed mold. Sample carved cartilaginous auricular framework on the left.

SINONASAL AND SKULL BASE SURGERY SIMULATORS

3D printing technology has been used in several areas of sinonasal and skull base simulation, mostly for educational use but also in work to assist surgical decision making. Manuel and colleagues[23] describe generating a 3D printed nasal model for use as a human nasal simulator to validate their finite element model of nasal tip deformity.

Their 3D printed construct used CT head data from a single patient and was produced in 2 components:

- Acrylonitrile butadiene styrene for the bony component
- Silicone soft tissue and cartilage component

The 3D printed so-called nasal phantom was then used as in its native and deformed states to validate a finite element model of nasal tip deformity. Ultimately the investigators hope that their finite element model will help quantify the highly subjective step in rhinoplasty planning of nasal tip palpation. If nasal tip palpation can be quantified and simulated, this may help improve rhinoplasty training, decrease the time to surgeon expertise, and diminish the importance of the unpredictable element of surgeon intuition.

Septoplasty/Rhinoplasty

Septoplasty is a procedure that is technically challenging to perform and difficult to both teach and learn because of the narrow endonasal workspace and complex and variable anatomy, as well as the inability of both the learner and the supervising surgeon to see while they are not directly performing the procedure.

AlReefi and colleagues[24] describe a novel 3D printed septoplasty simulator. They chose a patient CT with a moderate to severe deviation in septum anatomy, and printed in multiple materials to simulate differing tissue types:

- A rigid white opaque acrylic material, was used to print the bony construct.
- A rubberlike polymer, was used to print the skin and mucous membrane soft tissue elements.

These two commercially available 3D printing "inks" were combined to print and simulate the intermediate physical properties of cartilage. After several prototypes were printed and evaluated, the design was modified to include a layer of air bubbles between the mucosa and the bony-cartilaginous septum; this improved the fidelity of mucoperichondrial flap elevation.

Each model is single use, and the final prototype cost was $186 Canadian. In a large validation study, a cohort of 8 rhinologists, 6 senior residents, and 6 junior residents performed endoscopic septoplasty on the 3D printed trainer.

Participants completed a validation questionnaire assessing 3 domains:

- Realism, visualization, and educational impact
- Simulations were recorded and evaluated by 2 independent raters (single blinded)
- Postprocedure models were examined for performance metrics: quality, efficiency (time in minutes), and safety (eg, perforations)

The model showed reasonable fidelity and utility in training. Moreover, the investigators were able to detect a difference between the 3 groups of surgeons with respect to quality of procedure performed and efficiency, with more variable results for safety parameters. Although the quality and efficiency differences met statistical significance, the small group sizes warrant ongoing study to further validate this simulator.

Future directions for this group include consideration of making this model dynamic with the addition of bleeding to increase the fidelity of the procedural experience, as well as materials modifications, particularly with respect to coloration and removal of 3D printing support materials. Rhinoplasty is a complex surgical procedure that requires intricate soft tissue dissection skills to avoid injury to the cartilaginous framework. Furthermore, understanding the fundamental concepts of the structural integrity of the nose can be best appreciated by detailed examination of the anatomy.

Zabaneh and colleagues[25] developed a rhinoplasty simulator with 3D printed tools. Their model used 3D printed ABS (acrylonitrile butadiene styrene) plastic for the maxilla and nasal bones, and a series of molds manufactured on an inkjet printer. Molds were filled with various silicones to simulate the nasal cartilage as well as the mucosal layer and skin and soft tissue envelope. The construct was fully assembled and molded into a single-use construct. The investigators describe clear and opaque models for beginners and experienced learners but failed to describe any validation or objective outcomes. The cost of the simulator was not described; however, the investigators concluded that it has the potential to be used as a hands-on training module.

Endoscopic Sinus and Skull Base Surgery

Endoscopic sinus and skull base surgery relies heavily on the intraoperative use of CT and MRI for safe and effective surgery; many surgeons are now routinely using image guidance on complicated cases and/or for teaching. As such, 3D printing of this complex anatomic region seems a natural next step to facilitate training in this important area of the head and neck. Chan and colleagues[26] describe 2 endoscopic sinonasal simulators, one for sinus surgery training and the other for skull base training. Both are 3D printed using a cadaver's CT head data.

Sinus surgery trainer

The sinus surgery trainer is printed in acrylonitrile butadiene styrene. It eliminated turbinates and ethmoid sinuses to gain access to the nasal cavity and sinuses. Fiducial markers and peg features were added to allow for use of image guidance with the simulator. The simulator seems to be an examination model only at this time.

Investigators report that it is used for junior resident education of surgical anatomy and to teach endoscope handling. The print cost was approximately US$ 600. No validation data were reported; 3 surgeons reported qualitative assessments but only 1 surgeon's observations were reported.

Skull Base Surgery Trainer

The skull base surgery trainer is a bony construct printed in ZP-130 plaster powder (ZCorp, Burlington, MA); the cartilaginous elements in ZP-15 plaster are powered with elastomeric infiltrate applied to enhance compliance. No anatomic structures were eliminated, but the cartilaginous structures were slid into position (septum) or snapped into place (turbinates) within the bony construct. It was used to perform ethmoidectomy and surgical resection of the clivus with image guidance. The print cost was approximately US$900. A single surgeon assessed the model and gave qualitative feedback only; again, no validation studies are reported to date.

Endoscopic Endonasal Skull Base Drilling

Tai and colleagues[27] report an inexpensive, high-fidelity 3D printed model for endoscopic endonasal skull base drilling. It is printed using high-resolution patient maxillofacial CT and consists of skull frame printed in thermal plastic for durability, skull base drilling insert printed in an epoxy-coated plaster composite, and a skin and nasal cavity mask made from silicone that is molded by a 3D printed mold. Although the skull and skin mask are multiuse, the skull base drilling insert is single use.

The simulator features colored anatomic landmarks: carotid arteries, optic nerves/chiasm, pituitary, and so forth. The insert design may ultimately allow for patient-specific inserts to be 3D printed for surgical rehearsal, as well as to introduce other disorders, such as neoplasms, for training purposes. A model is used to perform sphenoidotomy, skeletonize carotids and sella turcica, and optic nerve decompression. The cost is approximately $500 for materials, and excludes 3D printer cost, as well as technical labor costs. The cost of the single-use insert was not reported.

Content validity was assessed in 5 domains by 8 neurosurgeons. Domains included physical attributes, realism of experience, value of simulator, relevance to clinical practice, and a global or overall rating. However, the small sample size allows modifications to be made and additional validation to be pursued thereafter. The model scored highest on value of the simulator, as reflected by agreement that the simulator has great potential as an educational tool. The model scored lowest on the global assessment, with expert raters largely agreeing that minor adjustments are needed before widespread use.

Future adjustments include anatomic modifications such as increased nostril size and softer nasal tissues, as well as more dynamic changes such as the implementation of bleeding to enhance surgical realism. Ongoing validation studies of alterations to the model are warranted, as are studies of educational impact on learners once the model is implemented in a curriculum.

LARYNGEAL SIMULATORS

Citing the need for airway procedural training in high-risk, low-frequency events, Kavanagh and colleagues[28] described the first 3D printed pediatric laryngeal simulators. These models simulate both normal anatomy and uncommonly encountered but challenging anomalies: laryngomalacia, subglottic stenosis, laryngeal cleft, and subglottic cysts.

The models were produced using 2 different 3D printing strategies:

- Direct 3D printed thin-walled plastic models
- Silicone elastomer (SE) models cast from 3D printed molds

The investigators designed a limited validation study to compare the models; 3 pediatric otolaryngologists and a single senior otolaryngology resident served as evaluators after using the models to perform:

- Direct laryngoscopy and bronchoscopy
- Suspension microlaryngoscopy procedures:
  - Supraglottoplasty, laryngeal cleft repair, and subglottic stenosis dilation

Both direct 3D printing and casting from a 3D printed mold result in highly anatomically accurate models of both normal and pathologic pediatric airway conditions. However, the assessments indicated that the tissue types of the models differed significantly in terms of procedural fidelity. The direct 3D printed models used the plastics polylactic acid, acrylonitrile butadiene styrene, and high-impact polystyrene; these were noted to be impossible or extremely difficult to manipulate surgically (ie, to incise, dilate, or suture).

The SE model was better suited to suspension direct laryngoscopy, as well as allowing for incisions and suturing. The SE models were slightly more expensive than the direct 3D printed models (US$6.85–6.97 vs US$2.08–4.71, respectively), which is an important factor in single-use models. This expense does not take into account the cost of 3D printers, or technical expertise costs.

In summary, this study is the first to describe 3D printed pediatric laryngeal models, as well as one of the few studies to date that has striven to 3D print disease states and pathologic anatomy for training purposes. Limited assessment of validation necessitates further study, at least in the SE model, because it seems to be a higher fidelity construct for future use. Educational impact is another area of further study.

Ainsworth and colleagues[29] also describe the use of 3D printing in developing a composite simulator for practicing transcervical laryngeal injection. They describe a 3D printed laryngeal framework and a variety of molded silicone soft tissue components that were used to help train residents in transcervical injection. They report improved comfort in residents who practiced on the simulator before patient experience.

FUTURE APPLICATIONS OF THREE-DIMENSIONAL PRINTING IN OTOLARYNGOLOGY

The utility of 3D printing in otolaryngology simulation has likely just begun to reveal its potential. Beyond trainee education, 3D printing may also have a role in patient-specific or disease-specific preoperative simulation for surgical rehearsal. A few reports have described the utility of a complex, case-specific simulator being used by an operative team to practice surgical approaches preoperatively.

Rose and colleagues[30] describe the use of a specific 3D printed temporal bone simulator for an 11-year-old patient with complex recurrent cholesteatoma. The multi-material model showed the disease extent and allowed the operative team to practice the surgical approach before the operation. The surgical team thought that it was subjectively useful.

Muelleman and colleagues[31] describe a case series of 3 patients with petroclival meningiomas who had 3D models generated of the lateral skull base tumor anatomy. Neurosurgeons and neurologists were then allowed to practice various middle fossa and posterior fossa approaches to the tumor before deciding on the best approach for each patient. The team reports that potential limitations in certain approaches were appreciated with the 3D models that had not been anticipated by the imaging alone, and they thought that these models were beneficial for the complex anatomy.

As 3D printing technology continues to improve, there is likely to be an impressive growth in patient-specific models for surgical rehearsal and simulation. In addition to temporal bone–specific models, this may also include anterior skull base disease, complex airway, and even robotic applications moving forward.

SUMMARY

3D printing is rapidly expanding across medicine, and has provided a novel approach for developing high-fidelity simulators and surgical trainers at low cost. To date, otologic and endoscopic simulators have predominantly been described because of the complexity of these surgical skills and the value in their simulation. It is anticipated that a wide variety of simulators across otolaryngology will be developed, and this will likely be supplemented by improvement in access and cost to the 3D printing technologies available. Patient-specific surgical rehearsal may have a significant role in this field for particularly complex disease or challenging exposure.

REFERENCES

1. Zopf DA, Hollister SJ, Nelson ME, et al. Bioresorbable airway splint created with a three-dimensional printer. N Engl J Med 2013;368(21):2043–5.
2. Mannoor MS, Jiang Z, James T, et al. 3D printed bionic ears. Nano Lett 2013; 13(6):2634–9.
3. D'Urso PS, Barker TM, Earwaker WJ, et al. Stereolithographic biomodelling in cranio-maxillofacial surgery: a prospective trial. J Craniomaxillofac Surg 1999; 27(1):30–7.
4. Gross BC, Erkal JL, Lockwood SY, et al. Evaluation of 3D printing and its potential impact on biotechnology and the chemical sciences. Anal Chem 2014;86(7): 3240–53.
5. Mitsouras D, Liacouras P, Imanzadeh A, et al. Medical 3D printing for the radiologist. Radiographics 2015;35(7):1965–88.
6. VanKoevering KK, Hollister SJ, Green GE. Advances in 3-dimensional printing in otolaryngology: a review. JAMA Otolaryngol Head Neck Surg 2016;143(2): 178–83.
7. Stansbury JW, Idacavage MJ. 3D printing with polymers: challenges among expanding options and opportunities. Dent Mater 2016;32(1):54–64.
8. Ventola CL. Medical applications for 3D printing: current and projected uses. P T 2014;39(10):704–11.
9. Raghunath N, Pandey PM. Improving accuracy through shrinkage modelling by using Taguchi method in selective laser sintering. Int J Mach Tool Manu 2007; 47(6):985–95.
10. Shirazi SF, Gharehkhani S, Mehrali M, et al. A review on powder-based additive manufacturing for tissue engineering: selective laser sintering and inkjet 3D printing. Sci Technol Adv Mater 2015;16(3):033502.
11. He Y, Xue GH, Fu JZ. Fabrication of low cost soft tissue prostheses with the desktop 3D printer. Sci Rep 2014;4:6973.

12. Suzuki M, Ogawa Y, Kawano A, et al. Rapid prototyping of temporal bone for surgical training and medical education. Acta Otolaryngol 2004;124(4):400–2.
13. Bakhos D, Velut S, Robier A, et al. Three-dimensional modeling of the temporal bone for surgical training. Otol Neurotol 2010;31(2):328–34.
14. Cohen J, Reyes SA. Creation of a 3D printed temporal bone model from clinical CT data. Am J Otolaryngol 2015;36(5):619–24.
15. Mowry SE, Jammal H, Myer CT, et al. A novel temporal bone simulation model using 3D printing techniques. Otol Neurotol 2015;36(9):1562–5.
16. Hochman JB, Kraut J, Kazmerik K, et al. Generation of a 3D printed temporal bone model with internal fidelity and validation of the mechanical construct. Otolaryngol Head Neck Surg 2014;150(3):448–54.
17. Mick PT, Arnoldner C, Mainprize JG, et al. Face validity study of an artificial temporal bone for simulation surgery. Otol Neurotol 2013;34(7):1305–10.
18. Da Cruz MJ, Francis HW. Face and content validation of a novel three-dimensional printed temporal bone for surgical skills development. J Laryngol Otol 2015;129(Suppl 3):S23–9.
19. Rose AS, Kimbell JS, Webster CE, et al. Multi-material 3D models for temporal bone surgical simulation. Ann Otol Rhinol Laryngol 2015;124(7):528–36.
20. Andrews JC, Mankovich NJ, Anzai Y, et al. Stereolithographic model construction from CT for assessment and surgical planning in congenital aural atresia. Am J Otol 1994;15(3):335–9.
21. Barber SR, Kozin ED, Dedmon M, et al. 3D-printed pediatric endoscopic ear surgery simulator for surgical training. Int J Pediatr Otorhinolaryngol 2016;90:113–8.
22. Berens AM, Newman S, Bhrany AD, et al. Computer-aided design and 3D printing to produce a costal cartilage model for simulation of auricular reconstruction. Otolaryngol Head Neck Surg 2016;155(2):356–9.
23. Manuel CT, Harb R, Badran A, et al. Finite element model and validation of nasal tip deformation. Ann Biomed Eng 2016;45(3):829–38.
24. AlReefi MA, Nguyen LH, Mongeau LG, et al. Development and validation of a septoplasty training model using 3-dimensional printing technology. Int Forum Allergy Rhinol 2016;7(4):399–404.
25. Zabaneh G, Lederer R, Grosvenor A, et al. Rhinoplasty: a hands-on training module. Plast Reconstr Surg 2009;124(3):952–4.
26. Chan HH, Siewerdsen JH, Vescan A, et al. 3D rapid prototyping for otolaryngology-head and neck surgery: applications in image-guidance, surgical simulation and patient-specific modeling. PLoS One 2015;10(9):e0136370.
27. Tai BL, Wang AC, Joseph JR, et al. A physical simulator for endoscopic endonasal drilling techniques: technical note. J Neurosurg 2016;124(3):811–6.
28. Kavanagh KR, Cote V, Tsui Y, et al. Pediatric laryngeal simulator using 3D printed models: a novel technique. Laryngoscope 2016;127(4):E132–7.
29. Ainsworth TA, Kobler JB, Loan GJ, et al. Simulation model for transcervical laryngeal injection providing real-time feedback. Ann Otol Rhinol Laryngol 2014;123(12):881–6.
30. Rose AS, Webster CE, Harrysson OL, et al. Pre-operative simulation of pediatric mastoid surgery with 3D-printed temporal bone models. Int J Pediatr Otorhinolaryngol 2015;79(5):740–4.
31. Muelleman TJ, Peterson J, Chowdhury NI, et al. Individualized surgical approach planning for petroclival tumors using a 3D printer. J Neurol Surg B Skull Base 2016;77(3):243–8.

Assessment of Surgical Skills and Competency

Nasir I. Bhatti, MBBS, MD

KEYWORDS

- Assessment • Surgical skills • Simulation • Competency • OSATS
- Formative feedback

KEY POINTS

- Objective Structured Assessment of Technical Skills (OSATS) is presently considered the "gold standard" for skills evaluation.
- Otolaryngology-specific OSATS have been developed and validated for many key index procedures.
- Faculty training through focused orientation sessions is critical for meaningful objective assessment.
- Timeliness of assessment and provision of formative feedback to residents enhance educational value of assessment systems.
- Crowd-sourced evaluations and mobile App technology are promising new methods that provide timely feedback with the potential to capture data across institutions.

Although operative skills represent only a part of the qualities needed to become a competent surgeon, the acquisition and assessment of these skills plays a central role in any surgical residency program. Over the past 2 decades, surgical educators have expressed concern over the perceived lack of confidence and competence among the graduating residents. This has led to increased interest in developing and using valid and reliable assessment systems, especially for measuring surgical competency.

Nevertheless, implementation of these systems into the day-to-day environment of surgical residency programs has been extremely difficult. Limited duty hours, restricted intraoperative autonomy, medico-legal and patient safety issues in addition to ever-increasing pressure on physicians' productivity are some of the leading challenges to training competent surgeons able to practice independently. Advocacy for more operative autonomy during residency is further complicated by the recent controversy over concurrent surgery in academic medical centers.

Disclosure Statement: The author has no commercial or financial conflicts of interest and there are no funding sources.
Johns Hopkins University, Department of Otolaryngology—Head and Neck Surgery, 600 North Wolfe Street, Baltimore, MD 21205, USA
E-mail address: Nbhatti1@jhmi.edu

Otolaryngol Clin N Am 50 (2017) 959–965
http://dx.doi.org/10.1016/j.otc.2017.05.007
0030-6665/17/© 2017 Elsevier Inc. All rights reserved.

oto.theclinics.com

Lack of faculty development programs for teaching faculty resulting in limited buy-in from them is another major impediment in implementing these assessment systems. The residency program directors have lamented about limited time, lukewarm support from the institutional leadership, and financial constraints as "missing pieces of the puzzle" in switching to competency-based medical education.

Residency programs are therefore seeking to create evaluation systems and to inculcate the culture changes needed to provide specific, timely, and consistent performance feedback to trainees to accelerate their progression toward operative competency and independent practice.

Defining Surgical Competency

Surgical competency may be defined as the ability to perform a task successfully producing desired results. Hall and colleagues[1] described surgical competence as an ability to successfully apply professional knowledge, skills, and attitudes to new situations as well as to familiar tasks.

Competency, as defined by Benner[2] in 1982, is a hierarchy that begins from novice, and goes through advanced beginner, competent, proficient, and finally to expert. Dreyfus and Dreyfus[3,4] also defined competency as a 5-stage model distributed into novice, competence, proficiency, expertise, and mastery. Although surgical competency can be defined in innumerable ways, it encompasses both technical and nontechnical skills.[5] Although the need for competence in technical skills for surgeons is self-evident, competence in nontechnical skills is increasingly being recognized as an important prerequisite for a safe surgeon. Hence, to attain competence, surgeons must develop not only technical skills but also nontechnical skills. The assessment systems used to measure surgical competence, therefore, need to incorporate tools to evaluate both technical and nontechnical skills explicitly, as well as implicitly.

Technical skills refers to psychomotor actions acquired via practice and learning related to the particular craft or field.[5] The collective term *nontechnical skills* has been used to describe behaviors encompassing situational awareness, decision making, team work, communication, and leadership. The association between nontechnical and teamwork skills and technical performance in the operating room is strong.[6-8] A vast majority of surgical errors, however, consists of technical mistakes, with more than half occurring due to a lack of competence.[9,10]

Assessing Surgical Competency

The introduction of the Modernizing Medical Careers framework in the United Kingdom along with the European Working Time Directive has significantly reduced the time allocated to train junior surgeons. A similar but less widely publicized situation exists in the General Surgery Residency environment in the United States. Before these changes went into action, a surgical trainee would log up to 30,000 working hours before becoming a consultant in the National Health Service. The Royal College of Surgeons estimated that these hours decreased significantly to 8000 hours and even further to 6000 hours with the implementation of Calman's proposal.[11] Therefore, there is a real need for these trainees to demonstrate their competency in operative skills to their faculty/peers by the end of their training programs. Similarly, in the United States, the Accreditation Council of Graduate Medical Education (ACGME) mandates that all surgeons graduating from residency training are competent to practice their surgical craft independently.

Recognizing the need to improve resident preparation for unsupervised practice, the ACGME, in collaboration with the American Board of Medical Specialties, launched the Outcomes Project in 2001.[12] The development of 6 core competencies thereafter was a major shift from the apprenticeship model that was previously used.[13] Evolution of the outcomes project led to transition to the New Accreditation System in 2012 that brought about the development of milestones. Experts in each specialty were given the task of developing milestones based on the competencies required for their residents to achieve for successful independent practice.[13]

Measuring operative competency in surgical specialties is an essential part of evaluating *Patient Care* (one of the ACGME core competencies). The development of milestones signifies a paradigm shift in graduate medical education as programs will be required to endorse not only experience but also competency in clinical and surgical performance.[13] The challenge of objectively and reliably assessing residents' surgical competence, however, has been well known to surgical trainers.[14] In a survey aimed at identifying the most important areas of research in surgical education, 9 of the top 10 research questions related to performance assessment and determination of achievement of competency.[15] This underlines the importance of development of new assessment and training tools while also highlighting the difficulty programs are facing with the proper implementation of the milestones-based assessments.

In response to this need and to stay compliant with the ACGME and ultimately the Milestones project of the individual residency review committees, many research groups reported on many novel methodologies and systems for surgical competency assessment. There was special emphasis placed on the need for providing timely formative feedback over the past 2 decades. Of the numerous assessment methods developed to evaluate surgical competency, Objective Structured Assessment of Technical Skills (OSATS) is presently considered the "gold standard" for objective skills assessment.[16,17] Other methods described to assess surgical competency include in-training examinations, 360-degree evaluations, index case analysis, surgical case logs, clinical exposure, and oral examinations of clinical practice.[14,18–26]

Table 1 lists various systems currently in use and compares them for efficiency, online availability, whether they can provide timely formative feedback, ease of use, and ability to assist with modular teaching. Most are limited in their ability to ensure that trainees receive personalized feedback in a consistent and timely manner, even while residents are increasingly being asked to provide operative performance assessments as a prerequisite for graduation. It is further alarming that very little objective data exist to guide competency-based decisions related to a resident. A few groups in otolaryngology head and neck surgery have reported development and validation of

Table 1
Comparison of surgical skills assessment systems

Assessment System	Efficiency	App-Based/ Online Availability	Formative Feedback	Feasibility	Modular Teaching	Objectivity
OSATS	**	**	***	**	***	*
OPRS	**	**	***	**	***	*
Simulation-based	*	*	**	*	***	**
SIMPL	***	***	**	***	**	*
Final product analysis	*	*	*	*	*	***
Eye-motion tracking	*	**	*	**	*	**

* low; ** moderate; *** high

Abbreviations: OSATS, Objective Structured Assessment of Technical Skills; SIMPL, system for improving and measuring procedural learning.

assessment tools based on the OSATS model. Lin and colleagues[14] reported development and validation of an objective assessment tool for endoscopic sinus surgery. Laeeq and colleagues[20] developed and tested a similar objective assessment tool for mastoidectomy. A significant body of work has been published on making these tools more feasible and generalizable for most of the surgical specialties. Despite a significant investment of time and resources, widespread usage of such tools remains an elusive target.

Current Challenges to Widespread Implementation

Work-hour restrictions for residents, and increasing demands for clinical productivity placed on faculty, requires the development of novel strategies for teaching and assessing operative skills.[16] Although development of new teaching and assessment methods is continuously in process, large-scale implementation of such systems and tools, along with the provision of timely feedback requires additional faculty time and resources, such as core materials and support personnel.[13] Hence, one of the biggest challenges in implementing any assessment system is faculty buy-in, as completion of assessment instruments at the end of an operative procedure puts an extra burden on faculty time.[13] In a nutshell, lack of time available to the attending surgeons results not only in low response rate on completing these evaluations but also a failure to provide timely formative feedback (**Box 1**).

Overcoming Challenges

In most residency programs, surgical skills are currently assessed at the end of rotation and generally consist of subjective faculty evaluations. Such subjective evaluations have proven to be recall-based and therefore carry poor reliability and validity.[13] To improve overall assessment and training of residents in surgical skills, the feedback should be timely and objective. To train residents for higher competencies under the new system, better defined learning objectives are also particularly important (**Box 2**). Although the development of milestones serves the purpose of objectively defining the training curriculum, complete implementation of all the milestones requires additional time and resources. Development of specific but feasible assessment tools is also required to evaluate the milestones. Different methods of skills assessment are appropriate in different situations.[18] As more and more residency training programs are embracing the milestones, new assessment tools pertinent to each program's requirements are being developed.

To address the issue of increased faculty time required for assessments, crowd-sourced evaluation of surgical skills has demonstrated promising results.[27–29]

Box 1
Barriers to implementing competency-based assessments

Service versus education

Work-hour restrictions

Greater demand for accountability

Additional time required for objective assessment and feedback

Reduced reimbursement for teaching activities

Lack of faculty buy-in

Increased program director workload

Box 2
Overcoming challenges of implementation
Better defined training objectives/milestones
Development of reliable assessment tools
Faculty development
App-based/crowd-sourced evaluations
Use of simulators
Nonphysician coaches to reduce faculty workload

Videotapes of resident performance were uploaded on the Internet and independent evaluators were asked to evaluate resident performance using predefined checklists. The evaluation provided by the independent evaluators had high correlation with faculty evaluations. Mobile Apps and technological advances offer the potential to address these issues by making it possible to collect "real-time" assessments for resident operative performances for all cases in which residents participated in the procedure.[30] The creation and wide adoption of such a system can potentially benefit not just at the individual and program levels, but also at the national level by providing an evidence base to set benchmarks for resident progression.

A major breakthrough in implementing an assessment tool has been published in a preliminary report from the procedural learning and safety collaborative in general surgery. A mobile application named system for improving and measuring procedural learning (SIMPL) has shown great promise in feasibility, buy-in from all stakeholders (residents, faculty, and programs).[31] The investigators believe that the system can provide data for measuring national trends in procedural learning for the residents. An added benefit is the dictated feedback that can augment surgical teaching by the attending surgeons. The most promising aspects of this project are ease of use, learning from sharing of lessons learned across institutions, and ability to generate enough assessment for each resident and from multiple evaluators for them to be meaningfully reliable. Initial success of this multi-institutional trial harbors well for similar efforts in other surgical specialties. One critical lesson from this report is the use of faculty development tools, such as orientation to the assessment tool and calibration of the evaluators by reviewing and comparing their assessments with others in the program.

In summary, assessment of surgical competency is undergoing a major paradigm shift. This has the potential to not only overcome the current challenges to surgical skills training but also provide opportunities to test novel interventions for making training more robust, efficient, and learner-centered. Novel AND feasible assessment tools would be used to guide resident learning, intraoperative teaching, and feedback by faculty and the provision of safe, progressive, operative autonomy to trainees.[31] Data collected from these assessments might help future educators get a better insight into the relationship between intraoperative resident autonomy, performance, and patient outcomes.

REFERENCES

1. Hall JC, Crebbin W, Ellison A. Towards a hybrid philosophy of surgical education. ANZ J Surg 2004;74:908–11.

2. Benner P. From novice to expert. Am J Nurs 1982;82:402–7.

3. Dreyfus S, Dreyfus H. A five stage model of the mental activities involved in directed skill acquisition. California University Berkeley Operations Research Center [monograph on the Internet]; 1980. Available at: http://www.dtic.mil/dtic/index.html. Accessed August 17, 2017.

4. Laeeq K, Waseem R, Weatherly RA, et al. In-training assessment and predictors of competency in endoscopic sinus surgery. Laryngoscope 2010;120:2540–5.

5. Ponton-Carss A, Kortbeek JB, Ma IW. Assessment of technical and nontechnical skills in surgical residents. Am J Surg 2016;212:1011–9.

6. Agha RA, Fowler AJ, Sevdalis N. The role of non-technical skills in surgery. Ann Med Surg (Lond) 2015;4:422–7.

7. Mitchell EL, Arora S, Moneta GL, et al. A systematic review of assessment of skill acquisition and operative competency in vascular surgical training. J Vasc Surg 2014;59:1440–55.

8. Alkhayal A, Aldhukair S, Alselaim N, et al. Toward an objective assessment of technical skills: a national survey of surgical program directors in Saudi Arabia. Adv Med Educ Pract 2012;3:97–104.

9. Meier AH, Gruessner A, Cooney RN. Using the ACGME milestones for resident self-evaluation and faculty engagement. J Surg Educ 2016;73:e150–7.

10. Holmboe ES, Call S, Ficalora RD. Milestones and competency-based medical education in internal medicine. JAMA Intern Med 2016;176:1601–2.

11. Chikwe J, de Souza AC, Pepper JR. No time to train the surgeons: More and more reforms result in less and less time for training. Brit Med J 2004;328(7437):418–9.

12. Accreditation Council for Graduate Medical Education. Milestones. Available at: http://www.acgme.org/What-We-Do/Accreditation/Milestones/Overview. Accessed August 24, 2016.

13. Brown DJ, Thompson RE, Bhatti NI. Assessment of operative competency in otolaryngology residency: survey of US program directors. Laryngoscope 2008;118:1761–4.

14. Lin SY, Laeeq K, Ishii M, et al. Development and pilot-testing of a feasible, reliable, and valid operative competency assessment tool for endoscopic sinus surgery. Am J Rhinol Allergy 2009;23:354–9.

15. Stefanidis D, Cochran A, Sevdalis N, et al. Research priorities for multi-institutional collaborative research in surgical education. Am J Surg 2015;209:52–8.

16. van Hove PD, Tuijthof GJ, Verdaasdonk EG, et al. Objective assessment of technical surgical skills. Br J Surg 2010;97:972–87.

17. Hopmans CJ, den Hoed PT, van der Laan L, et al. Assessment of surgery residents' operative skills in the operating theater using a modified Objective Structured Assessment of Technical Skills (OSATS): a prospective multicenter study. Surgery 2014;156:1078–88.

18. Ahmed A, Ishman SL, Laeeq K, et al. Assessment of improvement of trainee surgical skills in the operating room for tonsillectomy. Laryngoscope 2013;123:1639–44.

19. Francis HW, Masood H, Chaudhry KN, et al. Objective assessment of mastoidectomy skills in the operating room. Otol Neurotol 2010;31:759–65.

20. Laeeq K, Bhatti NI, Carey JP, et al. Pilot testing of an assessment tool for competency in mastoidectomy. Laryngoscope 2009;119:2402–10.

21. Barsuk JH, Cohen ER, Williams MV, et al. The effect of simulation-based mastery learning on thoracentesis referral patterns. J Hosp Med 2016;11:792–5.

22. Eppich WJ, Hunt EA, Duval-Arnould JM, et al. Structuring feedback and debriefing to achieve mastery learning goals. Acad Med 2015;90:1501–8.
23. Barsuk JH, Cohen ER, Potts S, et al. Dissemination of a simulation-based mastery learning intervention reduces central line-associated bloodstream infections. BMJ Qual Saf 2014;23:749–56.
24. Reh DD, Ahmed A, Li R, et al. A learner-centered educational curriculum improves resident performance on the otolaryngology training examination. Laryngoscope 2014;124:2262–7.
25. Wagner N, Fahim C, Dunn K, et al. Otolaryngology residency education: a scoping review on the shift towards competency-based medical education. Clin Otolaryngol 2017;42(3):564–72.
26. Brunt LM, Halpin VJ, Klingensmith ME, et al. Accelerated skills preparation and assessment for senior medical students entering surgical internship. J Am Coll Surg 2008;206:897–904 [discussion: 904–7].
27. Chen C, White L, Kowalewski T, et al. Crowd-sourced assessment of technical skills: a novel method to evaluate surgical performance. J Surg Res 2014;187:65–71.
28. Lodge D, Grantcharov T. Training and assessment of technical skills and competency in cardiac surgery. Eur J Cardiothorac Surg 2011;39:287–93.
29. Memon MA, Brigden D, Subramanya MS, et al. Assessing the surgeon's technical skills: analysis of the available tools. Acad Med 2010;85:869–80.
30. George BC, Teitelbaum EN, Meyerson SL, et al. Reliability, validity and feasibility of the Zwisch scale for the assessment of intraoperative performance. J Surg Educ 2014;71(6):e90–6.
31. Bohnen JD, George BC, Williams RG, et al. The feasibility of real-time intraoperative performance assessment with SIMPL (system for improving and measuring procedural learning): early experience from a multi-institutional trial. J Surg Educ 2016;73(6):e118–30.

Improving Team Performance Through Simulation-Based Learning

Mark S. Volk, MD, DMD

KEYWORDS

• Medical errors • Teamwork • Simulation based • Medical culture • SimZones

KEY POINTS

- An unacceptably large number of medical errors occur each year in US hospitals secondary to failure of adequate teamwork and communication.
- Development of good teamwork is impeded by the organizational, educational and cultural aspects of medicine. Unlike other high stakes industries, medicine seldom teaches or practices teamwork.
- Simulation-based team training is a means for health care practitioners to learn and practice teamwork principles such as crisis resource management.

Since construction of the first medical simulator in 1988 by Gaba and DeAnda,[1] simulation has become an increasingly valuable tool. Medical simulation now has diverse applications and is being used to train, prepare, and evaluate health care professionals as well as design policies and facilities for health care organizations. Perhaps the area in which it has the most potential impact is in improving teamwork among health care providers.

This article examines (1) the health care safety problem, (2) the barriers to teamwork in medicine, (3) improving health care teams using simulation-based team training, (4) developing a simulation-based teamwork training course, (5) the efficacy of simulation-based learning, (6) the future role of simulation-based teamwork learning in otolaryngology.

In discussing simulation-based learning and team performance the role of health care teams and how their function affects patient care must first be considered. For many years the health care industry has considered itself to be team oriented. Whether in the operating room (OR), the emergency room, or on patient floors, caregivers view themselves as part of a health care team. However, over the past 20 years the performance of these teams has been called into question.

Disclosure: The author has nothing to disclose.
Department of Otolaryngology and Communications Disorders, Boston Children's Hospital, 300 Longwood Avenue, Boston, MA 02115, USA
E-mail address: mark.volk@childrens.harvard.edu

Otolaryngol Clin N Am 50 (2017) 967–987
http://dx.doi.org/10.1016/j.otc.2017.05.008
0030-6665/17/© 2017 Elsevier Inc. All rights reserved.

THE SAFETY PROBLEM

There are currently significant safety problems within health care. These problems became widely evident with the publication of the Institute of Medicine (IOM) report in 1999.[2] The report stated that, because of medical errors, between 44,000 and 98,000 people each year die while inpatients in US hospitals. Subsequently, in 2000, Starfield[3] estimated that the number of deaths may be as high as 250,000 per year. In 2013, James[4] studied the same problem and found that the number is as high as 400,000 deaths per year. To put this into perspective, 400,000 deaths is the equivalent of four fully loaded commercial 747 airliner crashing every day for a year.[3,4] If this number of accidents were occurring in the airline industry it would have a profound effect on our society. Our faith in the safety of commercial flying would be shattered. Panic would ensue. Domestic and international travel and trade would come to an abrupt halt. These are the consequences of such a series of hypothetical disasters occurring in the airline industry.

However, a crisis of this magnitude is happening in health care. Despite being as deadly as the hypothetical airline catastrophe, the health care issues outlined earlier have a minimal impact on the public's perception of health care safety. In the airline industry every tragedy is in the news and publicly scrutinized and investigated, but in health care no such public scrutiny occurs. The health care safety problem is therefore under appreciated, even by health care providers.

As surgeons, otolaryngologists need to be particularly concerned regarding this epidemic because 66% of medical errors occur in the OR.[5] Of these errors, 54% are preventable.[6]

CAUSES OF HEALTH CARE ERROR

The causes of many health care errors are nontechnical. These are errors that occur not because of a lack of medical knowledge, preparedness, or technical ability; they occur because of a communication or teamwork breakdown. That is, the expertise to manage a crisis or clinical problem is usually at hand, but it is the ability of the health care team to organize, diagnose, plan treatment, and execute the treatment strategy that is often the stumbling block leading to most errors. Poor team performance accounts for the single most common cause of morbidity and mortality in health care. Several Joint Commission studies have shown that more than 60% to 70% of medical errors are secondary to teamwork and communication failures among clinicians.[7] In researching the cause of adverse events involving trainees, Singh and colleagues[8] showed that inadequate teamwork was responsible for 70% of 240 malpractice cases comprising mostly surgical residents. Poor team performance results in inefficiencies and poor patient outcomes, as well as tension and distress among staff.[9] Poor teamwork is the common denominator to most of the medical errors currently occurring. Despite this being known for some time, it appears that medical errors continue to occur at the same, or perhaps increasing, rates as in the past.[4,10,11]

BARRIERS TO TEAMWORK IN MEDICINE

Individuals inevitably make errors. The advantage of a high-performing team is that it identifies, resolves, and learns from the errors that are made by its individual members. Many of the barriers to good teamwork and communication in health care can be attributed to organizational, educational and cultural factors. Each of these elements has a synergistic effect in inhibiting good teamwork and communication.

ORGANIZATIONAL

Many of the team failures in health care are secondary to the organizational structure of those teams. Health care is inherently hierarchical. The health care unit in a typical teaching hospital consists of an attending, fellow, chief resident, intermediate resident, and junior resident and/or intern. Often there is a medical student as well. This hierarchy is seen on the wards, in the clinics, and especially in surgery. This situation produces a top-to-bottom form of communication. This communication style results in information being gathered and originating from the top, namely the attending, and being transferred, as deemed necessary, to the less senior members of the team. Some level of hierarchy is necessary and beneficial in bringing organization and planning to a team, but too steep a hierarchical gradient impedes communication. It tends to exclude the subordinate team members from participating in the diagnosis, treatment planning, and delivery of the patient care. Furthermore, subordinates are often deterred from alerting the rest of the team regarding potential errors in management and patient safety issues. This inhibition to speak up occurs because the social situation makes junior members of the team (junior residents, nurses) less comfortable with providing pertinent information and less likely to point out errors that they may perceive as happening. The juniors frequently think that everyone knows this information so they are intimidated and do not speak up. Often they fail to speak up to not look foolish or to avoid retribution. Such a situation was documented in an analysis of 50 pediatric residents' responses conducted by Landgren and colleaues.[12] This study surveys the reasons why residents on the floor fail to speak up regarding safety issues. The responses are shown in **Table 1**.[12] Reponses noted in the study that relate to factors such as intimidation, lack of communication, and a feeling of powerlessness are secondary to the hierarchical framework in which the residents work. Some of the responses reflect other pressures on teams, including production pressures (too busy caring for other patients, time constraints), lack of clinical skills (not sure whether I am right) or feeling that what might be said does not matter (knowing it will not go anywhere, no one will back you up). These examples are emblematic of what happens in many clinical settings. Note that the more senior house staff had a decreased percentage of these types of responses. This decrease demonstrates that inhibition to speak out lessens as trainees become more senior and increase in stature within the hierarchy.

Hierarchy is even more evident in the OR. A study by Sexton and colleagues[13] showed that 45% of surgeons tended to be supportive of a steep hierarchy within the OR compared with only 6% of intensive care unit (ICU) consultants and airline pilots supporting such a hierarchical structure in their work environments.[13] In the OR, the attending surgeon has traditionally had the role of the "captain of the ship". In this position, the attending surgeon has complete control of the surgical procedure and complete responsibility for the outcome of that procedure. This results in an accentuated hierarchy with an exacerbation of the organizational barriers discussed above.

EDUCATIONAL

The current lack of education in teamwork plays a significant role in reducing health care providers' ability to perform well in teams. This lack of education has an impact on safety in 2 ways. First, it prevents health care professionals from relating to each other and, second, it reduces health care providers' preparedness to handle emergencies. From the start of their training health care professionals train almost exclusively in silos and they rarely, if ever, train together. Nurses, physicians, and allied health providers all train in their own schools and fail to train together once they graduate.

Table 1
Reasons pediatric residents fail to speak up regarding safety issues

	Examples	Percentage of Respondents Listing Barrier (N = 93)
Perceived Personal Safety of Speaking Up		
Consequences of speaking up	Fear of hurting a professional relationship Being singled out for a systems-based error Fear of retaliation (eg, nurse not wanting to work with me)	9
Intimidation	People are more well liked if they do not serve as policemen Reminders responded to with signs, eye-rolling… There is a blame game, and I do not want to look like someone who raises issues too often and be seen as a troublemaker Too intimidated	9
Hierarchy	With certain attendings it is difficult to approach them Decisions made by superiors Afraid of the boss	9
Individual Factors		
Interpersonal skills	Embarrassment or humiliation Do not want to admit fault Unsure how to bring it up	13
Clinical skills	Assume attending experience outweighs my concerns Not sure whether I am right What I think might be a liability may not be one	9
Efficacy of Speaking Up		
Powerlessness	Nobody will back you up The feeling that nothing will get done It has already been spoken up about but nothing got done. So why bother again? Knowing it will not go anywhere	13
Contextual Factors		
Workload-related barriers	No time to appropriately speak up given a safety concern Time constraints Too busy caring for other patients	12
Motivation to Speak Up		
Uncertainty about event	Not being aware of an error Unsure whether truly an error	4
Concerns already addressed	Thinking someone else would do it Someone else probably reported it	2
No harm done	Error is not serious Does not seem like it would harm the patient	2

Residents were asked to list 3 barriers each, and so the percentages of residents listing each barrier do not add up to 100%.

From Landgren R, Alawadi Z, Douma C, et al. Barriers of pediatric residents to speaking up about patient safety. Hosp Pediatr 2016;6(12):740; with permission.

Personnel with various skill sets in aviation, utilities, the military, and symphony orchestras routinely train together so they can learn to work together. Health care is the only high-stakes industry that fails to educate their personnel in how to function as a team. It is therefore little wonder that teamwork during routine activities, and particularly during crises, is a cause of significant error. Not only do clinicians not conduct interprofessional team training but they rarely, if ever, train within their specialties to increase their preparedness. For instance, football teams practice 2-minute drills continuously throughout their season. The rationale is that they will be prepared to know what to do and to handle the pressure of needing to execute their plan with limited time at the end of the game. These teams practice their 2-minute drills so often that, when the time-pressured situation occurs in a game, they are able to perform as though it is a routine occurrence. In contrast, the same types of drills are never done in otolaryngology or any other surgical service. Because clinicians do not routinely practice (simulate) situations like airway emergencies or severe bleeding or an airway fire, their preparedness for performing optimally in these situations is diminished.

CULTURAL

The third aspect of medicine that adversely affects teamwork is cultural. As stated before, it is rare for medical students, nurses, respiratory therapists, and occupational therapists to train together. In addition to a lack of a shared fund of knowledge, this arrangement sets up a cultural hindrance to interprofessional teamwork. Weller and colleagues[14] discuss the various health care disciplines as tribes. Nurses, allied health professionals, physicians, and administrators all train separately and can all be considered as members of different tribes. In addition, because they undergo extensive postgraduate training, physicians are further split into various subtribes. Examples include surgeons, anesthesiologists, cardiologists, dermatologists, family practitioners, and intensivists. Because health care professionals are trained in their own silos, each professional group has a different educational background with a distinctly different knowledge base, manner of approaching problems, expectations on management of patients, and a unique way of communicating among themselves.[15] In short, each professional group, or tribe, has a different culture. The presence of this tribalism in medicine leads to a poor understanding of the roles, responsibilities and priorities of other members in multidisciplinary teams. Often members of one professional group fail to recognize the knowledge and skills of the other groups. Furthermore, this tribalism sets up a bias between tribes. Frequently members of one group tend to see qualities of their tribe as somehow more worthy than those of another.

OTHER FACTORS

There are other factors that are the basis for the team dysfunctions noted in health care. Many of these are secondary to the cultural factors previously mentioned. These factors include poor communication, lack of leadership, poor use of resources (both human and equipment), lack of role clarity, and inadequate global assessment. Of the teamwork elements listed earlier, the most important quality of high-functioning teams is good communication. In health care, communication most commonly breaks down in certain areas and under certain conditions, including handoffs during change of shifts, patient transfers between departments (eg, between otolaryngology and pulmonology) and locations (eg, OR to postoperative care), transfer of information between disciplines (eg, between doctors and nurses), and in high-acuity settings such as the emergency room or in surgery.

THE OPERATING ROOM: A SPECIAL ENVIRONMENT

It is not surprising that the OR is the area with the highest number of medical errors. Lingard,[9] in a study of 48 surgical procedures spanning 90 hours, showed that 30% of communications failed to convey the intended information and 10% of those communications resulted in adverse effects ranging from inefficiencies and team tension to delays and procedural errors. When a crisis occurs in a clinical setting the need for good teamwork increases but the ability to function as a high-performance team is reduced. Mazzocco and colleagues[16] showed that surgical outcomes are linked directly to the teamwork and cooperation of the operative team. Nagpal and colleagues[17] showed that vital information from the anesthesia/surgery team was often not conveyed to the ward nurses caring for postoperative patients on the floor. Essential operative/anesthetic information was relayed only 67% of the time. Vital information on the patients' allergies (55%), comorbidities (30%), blood loss (20%), and significant surgical events (15%) was successfully imparted to the postoperative nursing service even less frequently.[17] All of this is not unexpected given that the OR is a virtual "perfect storm" for breakdown in communication and teamwork. Factors that are often present in the OR and that contribute to such a breakdown include[18]:

- Time pressure (production/scheduling issues as well as the acute nature of surgical emergencies)
- Frequent rotation of OR personnel (on a day-to-day basis as well as during the course of each day)
- The presence of multiple services (surgery, anesthesiology, and nursing)
- Participation by trainees
- A definite, steep hierarchy

THE ATTRIBUTES OF A HIGH-PERFORMANCE TEAM

Brannick and colleagues[19] defined a team as "two or more individuals who work together to achieve specified and shared goals, have task-specific competencies and specialized work roles, use shared resources, and communicate to coordinate and to adapt to change."

These objectives seem to be fairly easy to achieve. However, because of the organizational, educational and cultural barriers mentioned earlier, health care providers often work in a culture and an environment that makes it difficult for them to fulfill these criteria. For instance, as stated earlier, an essential aim of a team is to have a shared goal. Even this basic objective may be difficult to attain in the health care setting. One of the reasons for this is that, based on divergent training, members of an interdisciplinary team perceive a problem differently because they lack common backgrounds. In addition, if they agree on a common goal (eg, need to stabilize the airway), they may have very different ideas and expectations as to how to attain the goal given their different experiences on how to treat such a problem. This lack of common training before a crisis is then compounded by poor interdisciplinary communication during the crisis.

IMPROVING TEAMWORK IN HEALTH CARE

Medicine is a high-pressure, high-stakes activity. There is often significant time pressure and it requires a high level of expertise and resources. Poor performance results in harm or even death to the patient. There are several other industries that share these high-pressure, high-stakes characteristics. These industries include the railroads, the military, and nuclear power. However, many of these industries have superb safety records. It is useful to explore how these industries that function in similar conditions as medicine have been able to produce such an admirable safety record. One of the best and most well-studied examples of a high-pressure, high-stakes industry is aviation. It has many parallels with medicine.

During the mid–twentieth century, aviation had safety issues. These issues seemed to be related to poor team performance, which came to light in the late 1970s when the National Transportation Safety Board (NTSB) began including psychologists as part of the crash investigation teams. Perfectly flight-worthy aircraft were crashing at an alarming rate. The aircraft were crashing not because they were malfunctioning. They were not crashing because the pilots were making flying errors. Instead, they were crashing because of team and communication failures. Three examples of this type of failure come to mind: (1) the Tenerife disaster, in which a 747 captain mistakenly thought he had takeoff clearance and proceeded down a foggy runway and struck another aircraft on the ground[20]; (2) Eastern flight 401, in which the crew neglected to actively fly the plane because they were distracted by a light bulb that failed to illuminate, leading to a gradual loss of altitude and the crashing of the aircraft[21]; (3) United Airlines flight 173, in which a burned out light bulb distracted the captain and caused him not to respond to warnings regarding low fuel levels. The plane ran out of fuel in midair and crashed.[22] The pilots who were flying these planes were technically very competent. However, from reviewing the flight voice recorders from these and numerous other crashes, it became apparent that many of the failures were not caused by the pilots' technical skills. Instead, most mishaps occurred secondary to other factors, such as poor leadership, not speaking up, failure to allocate resources, and/or loss of situational awareness.

These examples exemplify the types of errors associated with teamwork failure. Similar teamwork errors are typical of those currently occurring in health care.

PRINCIPLES AND SIMULATION

It became apparent from these and other disasters that improving teamwork and communication was the key to improving airline safety. It was at that time that United Airlines developed a set of principles, cockpit resource management. These principles addressed many of the issues with which flight crews were struggling. However, developing a set of principles was not enough. The principles were taught and practiced using an experiential learning tool, namely simulation. Because aviation was already using flight simulators, scenarios were developed for the flight simulator that enabled crews to learn and practice cockpit resource management. With the use of simulation, cockpit resource management principles rapidly became part of the training of virtually all commercial airline pilots worldwide. With almost all pilots being trained in cockpit resource management principles, many of the previous errors started to become eliminated. At about the same time the number of airline disasters decreased precipitously. Note that during this time several safety measures were simultaneously being adopted in aviation so the effect of cockpit resource management on this improvement in safety is unclear.

By adhering to cockpit resource management principles, aviation crew members were able improve their cooperative efforts and their team performance. These principles also facilitated a change in aviation culture. The attitude toward error changed. Previously the concept of error revolved around the ideal of all error being intolerable and secondary to individual failure. The person who made an error was subject to recrimination. With cockpit resource management this notion changed. It became accepted that human error is inevitable and that an error-free system is not possible. Likewise, individuals are often blind to the errors they make.[23] With this as the working theory, the role of team members evolved so that each individual was on alert for errors that they or other members of their team will inevitably make. By the same token, errors were studied in the open so that they became topics for learning rather than recrimination. To encourage this, even the structure of error reporting was changed. Errors used to be conveyed to the Federal Aviation Administration (FAA), the agency that certifies pilots. This system tended to bring out about a punitive aspect to the process. This process was changed so that errors reports went to the National Aeronautics and Space Administration (NASA), where they were embraced and studied as means to bring about improvement.

Flying an aircraft and taking care of an ill patient are distinctly different endeavors, but they have some important similarities when it comes to team performance. Aviation was able to overcome its teamwork problem and so it made sense to pattern medicine's teamwork remediation strategies after those in the airline industry.

SIMULATION IN HEALTH CARE

Simulation is an experiential educational tool that has many applications in health care. These range from simple skills simulators to complex multidisciplinary simulations. Simulation may be used to educate trainees, assess performance, develop processes and protocols and assist in medical facility design. When most people think of medical simulation, a skills type simulator usually comes to mind. Otolaryngologists have been longtime users of temporal bone labs during residency training. Temporal bone dissection is essentially a skills simulator for ear surgery. Other skills simulators include Resusi-Annie for cardio-pulmonary resuscitation training and an intravenous (IV) placement simulator to teach IV access. These examples are simple but skills simulators may be elaborate. For example, they can be used to teach laparoscopic surgery or extracorporeal membrane oxygenation cannulation to novices and intermediates. Experts may also use them to hone their previously acquired skills. No matter what the level of sophistication, the purpose is straightforward: to teach trainees a specific skill.

As on progresses beyond skills simulators, the simulation is tailored depending on the level of the participant/trainees. In transitioning from novice to expert, both the signal/noise ratio of the simulation and the degree of active, hands-on teaching decrease. Roussin and Weinstock[24] classified simulation in health care into 4 zones, depending on the expertise of the participants and the educational goal of the simulation (**Fig. 1**). Using an IV insertion simulator is a skills simulation in zone 0. Here simulation is being used to teach a basic technique. There is not much in the way of extraneous clinical information or extraneous distractions. There is no ambiguity to the participant as to what needs to be accomplished during the simulation. The instructor is with the trainee the whole time. The instructor takes a hands-on approach and may verbally or even physically guide the trainee during the exercise. The simulation is paused as many times as necessary to make a teaching point or to allow the participant to ask questions. When the trainee reaches the goal (gets the IV started) the trainee knows this and obtains automatic feedback. During this skills session the questions being asked are why and how is the procedure being done. The participant is being continually given feedback and debriefed during the simulation. Moving to the higher zones on the right, the signal increases in amount and complexity. The simulations become more intricate and realistic. There is more distraction as the complexity and ambiguity of the information increase. Just as in a real-life situation, it becomes more difficult to determine which information is important and which is extraneous.

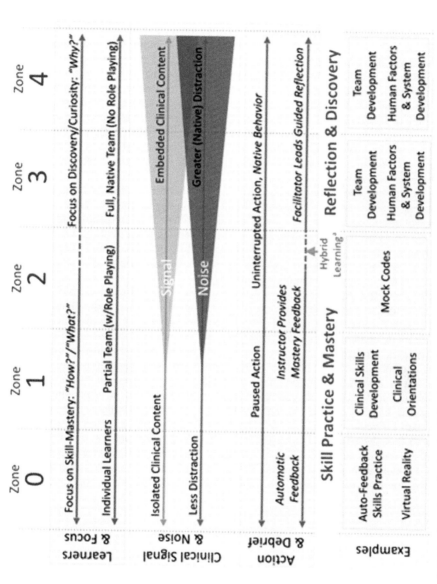

Fig. 1. SimZones. A means to categorize levels of simulation. (*From* Roussin CJ, Weinstock P. SimZones: an organizational innovation for simulation programs and centers. Acad Med 2017;92(8):1114–20; with permission.)

Team training is usually done in zone 2 or zone 3. In these zones of simulation, the scenarios can be quite realistic. Zone 2 is usually performed with a partial clinical team, with the other members of the team comprising actors or simulation personnel role playing. Simulation in zone 3 involves full, native teams. That is, there is a full complement of team members who often work together. Because there is a full complement of clinicians, there is no role playing. Zones 2 and 3 are also called high-fidelity simulation. This type of simulation involves a sophisticated manikin. These manikins have various capabilities. In general, they are able to talk (through a speaker with the help of a simulation technician), their chest walls move with respiration, and they may have pupils that can contract or dilate. The degree of interaction with the instructors/facilitators during the simulation is minimal. The instructors are there only to answer the occasional question about clinical findings on the manikin and to troubleshoot any issue with the simulation scenario. They do not advise or help the participants during the simulation, and the simulation proceeds without interruption until the end of the scenario. At that point there is an extensive debrief. During these debriefs, the purpose is not to determine what or how something needs to be done. The goal is to determine why something happened or why someone was motivated to act in a certain way.

At present, the bulk of learning during postgraduate medical education is through the clinical experience that physicians receive while taking care of patients. The concept of see one, do one, teach one is still operative. This concept is starting to change in fields such as general surgery in which trainees must attain a certain level of technical skill on the simulator before doing actual laparoscopic surgery. As mentioned earlier, a simulated training situation, temporal bone dissection, has been in place for many years in otolaryngology.

In comparing the experiential learning environment of an actual clinical experience versus a simulated experience, medical simulation has some advantages (**Table 2**). In actual practice, clinical experiences are random and depend on luck regarding what and how many cases or conditions a resident see during residency. This situation is unlike medical simulation, in which training programs can guarantee exposure to certain clinical situations. Feedback after a real clinical encounter is haphazard, whereas it is always a component of a simulated experience. As far as realism goes, an actual event is, of course, the real thing. In a simulated environment the realism varies from low-fidelity to high-fidelity simulation, to situations in which the events can be super-real. Super-real simulation occurs when events can be juxtaposed so that they have a learning effect that almost never occurs in real life. An example of this is a simulated case of a tension pneumothorax followed by a simulation of a patient with a bronchial cast. Presenting them in successive simulations allows the trainees to compare the clinical features of these two conditions. In

Table 2
Educational properties of actual versus simulated clinical events

	Actual Clinical Event	Simulated Clinical Event
Nature of experience	Few, unstructured, uncontrolled	Possibly many, structured, controlled
Feedback	Uncommon	Always
Realism	As real as it gets	Low fidelity to high fidelity to super-real
Errors	Potential harm to patient (and caregiver?)	Valuable part of learning

addition, error is viewed differently in real versus simulated occurrences. Error is something to avoid during a real patient encounter because it leads to safety issues for the patient and possible psychological consequences for caregivers. In contrast, errors are embraced in simulation and are used as teaching points.

SIMULATION-BASED TEAM TRAINING

As previously discussed, aviation crews use simulators to learn and practice cockpit management principles so they are able to use these principles in both routine and crisis situations. Similarly, the purpose of providing simulation-based training to health care providers is to enable them to learn and practice teamwork principles. The teamwork principles that are being used in health care are derived from the airline industry and are know as crisis resource management principles or CRM. The 5 principles of CRM for health care are listed in **Box 1**. Teamwork is taught within the framework of these principles.

BUILDING A SIMULATION-BASED TEAMWORK TRAINING COURSE
Organizational Planning

Just as preparation and planning are essential to good clinical practice outcomes, careful planning is needed to launch a successful simulation-based teamwork training course. Most simulation courses designed to teach teamwork are usually at a zone 3 level or are hybrids in zone 2. They can be single specialty but, for the reasons delineated earlier, they are more effective if they are multidisciplinary.

The first step in developing a course is to determine the groups and the training levels for which the course is targeted. Because most teamwork courses in surgery are targeted toward the surgical team, this means surgeons (otolaryngologists), nurses, and anesthesiologists. However, it could involve ICU and or emergency department personnel as well. The participants' level of training also needs to be taken into account. Usually these courses involve multilevel teams, such as 1 or 2 residents of different training levels headed by either a fellow or an attending. In order to recreate realistic hierarchies, there should be equivalence between the medical specialties. Therefore, it makes sense to avoid asymmetrically composed teams, such as an anesthesia group headed by an attending and an Otolaryngology team whose senior member is a fellow. The nursing team is usually composed of nurses of different seniority/experience.

Producing a simulation-based teamwork course in itself often requires extensive teamwork and coordination. Once the disciplines and level of the course participants are determined, it is essential to enlist champions from each of the discipline's constituencies. These committed individuals act as collaborators in planning the course. They have the ability to lend their specialty's perspectives in developing course

| Box 1 |
| The 5 principles of crisis resource management |
| Role clarity |
| Communication |
| Personnel support |
| Resource allocation |
| Global assessment |

learning objectives. This is necessary to provide course content that is relevant to each clinical group. Early in the course development process these colleagues are often invaluable in "selling" the course to their respective departments and department administrations. As the course becomes operational, they function as codirectors and are helpful as ongoing course liaisons, advocates, and troubleshooters. Having champions within each of the participating departments helps enable personnel scheduling for the course. Ideally, they should help run the course and act as facilitators for the course debriefings.

Concurrently with all this, it is important to involve your institution's simulator program personnel. They are a good source of ideas and can suggest and advise you on the possibilities and feasibility of your plan. They can also start to brainstorm with you on the educational goals and objectives as well as the course structure.

Simulation Location

One of the first things to determine when contemplating simulation-based team training is the physical environment in which the simulation scenarios will occur. Because of the large number of real-life errors that occur in the OR and the presence of multiple specialties (surgeons, anesthesiologists, and nurses), it is a simulated environment that lends itself to producing scenarios that are engaging to all participants. Other possible sites are the emergency department, a patient's room on the floor, or an ICU. The simulations may be done in a simulation center, or they may be done in situ at the clinical point of care.[18,25] Both a simulation center and a point-of-care location have their own advantages and disadvantages. Holding simulations in a simulation center is less expensive because they do not use clinical space with the resulting loss of clinical revenue. Also, simulations performed in a simulation center prevent the possibility of the simulation interfering with patient care. In situ simulations have the advantage of increased realism (the setting does not just look like an OR, it is an OR). Because these simulations occur at the point of care, the clinicians are already located in close proximity to the simulation site. They do not have to travel across town or across the street to access the simulation center. There is no right or wrong answer as to which location is best. It depends on an institution's facilities, resources, and preferences.

Administration Support

Before attempting a simulation-based course it is important to obtain buy-in from all the involved parties. For a multidisciplinary OR simulation course it is essential that assent and cooperation be obtained from all parties. This process may include hospital administration; OR administration; the simulation program; and the nursing, anesthesia, and surgery (otolaryngology) departments. Contacting these individuals along with the pertinent specialty champion to discuss the course plans is essential. Here is where your colleagues from the involved disciplines can be very helpful. You, the specialty-specific colleague, and perhaps a representative from the simulation program need to meet with and inform the department head of the preliminary course objectives and plans. Make them aware of what resources may be needed to bring the course to fruition. They need to be made aware of and sign off on the estimated time, personnel, and funding required for the course. It is important to do this early on rather than discover a serious obstacle from one of the participating groups later in the process. The need for team training and the benefits of simulation-based training are becoming more accepted but there remain skeptics. Securing acceptance for your course may take some convincing. You may want to bring along a short presentation to highlight the needs for teamwork and the benefits of your proposed course. If needed, offer to make your presentation to the department as a group.

Course Development

Once the planning team has come together, the objectives of the course have been delineated, and the administrative approval has been obtained, specific course planning and development may occur. In general, simulation-based teamwork training courses tend to have 3 components: didactics, simulation, and debriefing. Use of these components is theoretically sound because it is supported by the Kolb Learning Cycle, an adult learning theory.[26] This theory states that adults learn in a continuum of experience, reflection, conceptualization, and experimentation. The 3 simulation teaching components work synergistically within Kolb's[26] theoretic framework (**Fig. 2**).

Time is a valuable commodity in health care. It may be challenging for the most dedicated team members to break away from clinical activities and attend a simulation session. Because of this, one of the most difficult aspects of running a successful simulation course is scheduling. Be aware of the significant planning issues that exist around scheduling clinicians from multiple departments as participants. Make sure that your facilitators are available. Realize that the simulator, OR, and clinical space (if needed) and conference room space are often at a premium and need to be booked ahead of time. Work closely with your champions from other departments and the simulator program arrange for available space and personnel ahead of time. Think ahead. These courses need to be booked 6 to 12 months in advance.

Simulation courses have many components, so practice what you preach and run pilot simulation scenarios to work out the kinks before your first course. If you are not able to run a pilot course, let the participants of the first course know that this is a pilot and that it may not go as smoothly as you hoped. Invite feedback from them on how it may be improved.

Didactic

Simulation courses usually start with a didactic portion. This allows the participants to be greeted, gives them an idea of the purpose of the course, and orients them to the simulation/debriefing process. Additional didactic material may be presented between simulation scenarios.

Most courses start with introductions. Going around the room, the participants and faculty members introduce themselves, say what their roles are in the hospital (eg, OR nurse, third year, otolaryngology resident), describe their experience in simulation, and

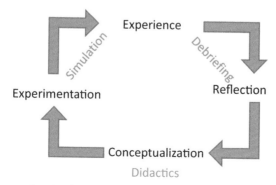

Fig. 2. The elements of a simulation course (didactics, simulation, debriefing) overlaid on the foundations of Kolb Learning Theory.

provide an "icebreaker." The icebreaker involves each person answering a standard question about themselves in order for the participants to relax and get to know each other. The question is usually a simple one, such as what is their favorite food is, or their favorite place where they have traveled.

Many participants, especially those encountering simulation for the first time, approach simulation with significant anxiety. For many of them it is a high-stakes endeavor. Unlike a clinical situation, the stakes are high not based on the outcome of the patient but on the perception of the participants that they will be scrutinized or judged harshly. It is important to place them at ease early. Most simulationbased teamwork training courses are nonevaluative. It is critical to inform the participants of this early in the didactics. They need to know that they will not be given a grade or evaluated in any way. Perhaps most importantly they need to know that the course is all about learning and sometimes the best lessons are learned from mistakes.

At this juncture, the confidentiality of the simulation is reviewed. Because the scenarios work best if their content is not known beforehand, we ask the participants not to discuss the details of the simulations to anyone after the simulation course. As part of the nonevaluative nature of the simulation, everyone (instructors and participants) is requested not to discuss individual performances to anyone after the simulation course is concluded.

Next is an orientation to the simulation environment. This orientation is an instructional talk on what to expect during the simulation. Participants are told that their role is to act as they normally would during the clinical situation. Thus, PGY-2 anesthesia residents should act as themselves during the scenarios. In orienting the participants to the manikin, they are told where to listen for breath sounds, where to palpate for pulses, and what kind of procedures are permitted. Depending on the type of manikin, these usually include intubation, chest tube placement, cricothyroidotomy, tracheostomy, bronchoscopy, and esophagoscopy. They are told what equipment is available, what drugs they can use, what to do if they are unsure of their exam of the manikin and how to call a code if the manikin arrests.

Simulation Scenario Design

The heart of any simulation-based course is the simulation itself. In designing a scenario the following elements must be kept in mind:

1. The scenario needs to be plausible to the participants. The scenario cannot seem to be arranged or far-fetched. The facts and progression of the scenario must fit together in a cogent, logical manner. One of the best ways to develop such a scenario is to use or adapt an actual case, such as one that may have been presented at a morbidity and mortality conference. Using an actual previous case ensures that patient's history, physical findings, and outcome are all consistent with a real situation. In introducing the scenarios to the participants, try to be as informative as possible regarding the case, its history, and the resources available to the participants. If it is important that the participants know that the manikin has a drug allergy, state it clearly at the beginning of the scenario or make sure it is written prominently in the chart. Do not introduce contrived elements, such as equipment failure (Bovie or head light not working), power outages, or resource shortages (eg, claiming that "radiology can only take 1 more radiograph").
2. The scenario should have elements that engage as many of the course participants as possible. For example, in a multidisciplinary scenario that involves nurses, surgeons, and anesthesiologists, it is important that the manikin develops both a surgical and an anesthesia/medical problem. This will make it more likely that each participant

will be engaged. In otolaryngology simulations, this is fairly simple because any scenario with an airway issue simultaneously challenges both the surgeons and the anesthesiologists. Airway scenarios may also be challenging for nursing staff because these situations often require the nurse to expeditiously procure and set up a significant amount of equipment, such as bronchoscopes and tracheotomy sets.

3. The subject matter and the difficulty of the scenario need to coincide with the abilities of the participants. When developing scenarios, it is important to be aware of the participants, their knowledge/skills, and their experience. As an example of this, a case in which the patient has a hemorrhaging tracheal tumor may not be an appropriate scenario for a group of solely otolaryngology residents but might be perfect for a team that includes cardiothoracic trainees. Just because a group of participants has never seen the type of case portrayed in the scenario does not mean that it would not be appropriate for them. On the contrary, simulation is perfect for enabling practitioners to encounter and practice managing well-known but uncommon emergency situations. Examples of these include an airway fire or a postthyroidectomy hematoma. Most otolaryngologists know what to do in these situations, but they rarely, if ever, have the opportunity to contend with and manage them (**Fig. 3**).

4. Scenarios need to be developed that fit within the time frame of the simulation course. They can be as short as 5 to 10 minutes or as long as 45 minutes. The educational purpose of the scenario is to allow the participants to practice teamwork. During the course of the scenario the facilitators who will be leading the debriefing take note of examples of good and less-than-desirable aspects of the team's behaviors. Once they think that they have collected enough behavior examples to allow a good discussion during the debriefing, then the scenario can be ended. It takes some experience to gauge how long a scenario needs to run before the educational goals are met. Often, if the participants in the scenario are at the point at which they are about to achieve their clinical goal, such as securing an airway, retrieving a foreign body, or establishing a diagnosis, then they are allowed to continue.

5. The scenarios used for team training are designed to illustrate and teach team principles. This is frequently done by down playing the medical features of the scenarios and accentuating the teamwork aspects. To do this, the scenarios usually have relatively simple medical management concepts. But, while the medical

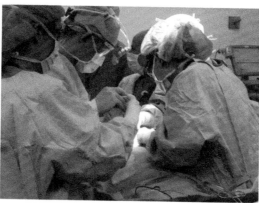

Fig. 3. High-fidelity, in situ, multidisciplinary team training simulation. Participants are managing an intraoperative tracheostomy emergency.

"solution" is straightforward, the scenario has a crisis quality brought about by an acute deterioration in the patient's condition. This emergency environment brings out the teamwork issues within the participant group. These then can be used during the debriefing to demonstrate and impart teamwork principles.

An example of this would be the case of a patient who presents to the Emergency Room after accidental decannulation. As the patient's clinical condition starts to deteriorate, the physicians (Otolaryngology, Anesthesia and Emergency Medicine) and the nurses need to determine what to do and how best to accomplish the task of restoring a stable airway. The theoretical solution of reestablishing an airway is simple. But, the teamwork problems that arise in this setting can be both quite challenging and educational.

6. The desired degree of urgency of the scenario is best achieved by titrating the severity and acuity of the patient's condition. The severity level can best be accomplished by altering the manikin's vital signs, level of consciousness, stridor, skin color, etc. The acuity is controlled by the rate at which these clinical signs and symptoms deteriorate.

Realism

The purpose of the simulation scenarios is to engage the learners so that they at some level perceive the scenario as real. This engagement allows them to think, act, and interact with their team members in a realistic manner. Then, during the postsimulation debriefing, the facilitators, along with the participants, review the events during the scenario. Within the framework of the CRM principles they then discuss why those actions occurred and how they can be improved to promote better teamwork in the future.

The scenarios only need to have a level of realism that allows participant engagement. The degree of realism needed to achieve the scenario's objective usually depends on the level and experience of the participants. Experts or more experienced participants, such as attending surgeons and anesthesiologists, often require a more sophisticated simulation compared with residents or medical students. An example of this is a scenario designed for residents and fellows that deals with teamwork issues involving intraoperative complications of tracheostomy tube placement. The trainees are tasked with placing a tracheostomy during which the patient has complications. In this scenario, the manikin's tracheal anatomy is rudimentary and not lifelike. However, because the trainees become engaged by the clinical situation, namely the intraoperative complications, it does not register with them that the tracheostomy procedure is unrealistic. Because the objective of the exercise is to examine the teamwork issues associated with the complications and not to teach tracheostomy tube placement, the reduced realism of this aspect of the scenario does not affect its educational goals. This same scenario would likely not be successful with attending otolaryngologists because this reduction in realism to a group of more expert participants would result in a lower level of engagement.

Debriefing

In simulation there is a saying that simulation is an excuse to debrief. In many ways the debriefing is the most important part of the simulation session. Immediately after the scenario is finished the participants are asked to proceed to a conference room for the debriefing, which starts as soon as possible. A debriefer and a codebriefer facilitate the debriefing session. Often they are also facilitators from the scenario. Both are trained in debriefing techniques. One of the debriefing team may or may not be a medical clinician. This person could be a psychologist, a medical educator, or a clinician from another field of medicine. One of the debriefers is usually someone who has medical expertise in the simulated case, such as an otolaryngologist, an anesthesiologist, or a nurse. In addition to helping with the debriefing of the teamwork issues, this person also acts as a content expert for the medical aspects of the scenario.

The debriefing sessions have a 3-phase structure. At the beginning of the debriefing the debriefer explains the structure of the session. The debriefer also lets the participants know that, in virtually all simulations, there are errors. One of the purposes of the debriefing is to embrace these errors, use them as teaching points, and learn from them. The first phase in the debriefing is the reaction phase. During this segment the participants are encouraged to share with each other how they felt emotionally. This phase allows them to vent about the scenario that they just experienced. Often the comments made by the participants in this phase give clues to issues that might be explored later on. An example is a nurse who says "I was so frustrated, I kept going out of the room to get stuff but I never knew why I was getting it." This type of comment might trigger a discussion later in the debriefing about the advantages of having everyone aware of the patient's clinical condition and interventions that are being contemplated. The next phase of the debriefing is the understanding phase. This phase is the main substance of the debriefing, and has 2 parts. The first is the discussion of the medical issues involving the simulated patient. In this portion of the debrief the group discusses the diagnosis and condition of the simulated patient (eg, a large foreign body in the esophagus causing tracheal compression and respiratory distress) and the treatment (eg, bronchoscopy followed by esophagoscopy). During the second part of the understanding phase the participants are asked as a group, and as individuals, questions about behaviors observed by the facilitators during the scenarios. The point of this part of the exercise is to examine a behavior (eg, inability to speak up), discuss how it affects teamwork (eg, valuable information lost to the team), and then find out why that person acted in that manner (eg, intimidated, afraid they were wrong, thought everyone else was already aware of what might have been said). Then that behavior is generalized into the context of other participants' experiences (eg, whether anyone else has done this or felt this way). This shared experience is put into the context of the CRM principles (in this case, communication and role clarity). In addition, the group explores possible ways in which a similar, real situation may best be handled in the future. The debriefers then select 1 or 2 other issues and go through a similar process. The last phase of the debriefing is the summary phase. As would be expected, the debriefer presents a summary of some of the issues discussed, the CRM principles involved, and some possible solutions that the group has been able to formulate.

During the debriefing the debriefers attempt to draw the participants out, offer suggestions, and guide them to what it is hoped are helpful solutions. The purpose is to make the participants aware of the teamwork issues involved in the scenarios. The experiences that they have in the simulator and the debriefings tend to have a powerful impact. Often participants are amazed at how difficult it can be to work effectively together as a team. It is hoped that, over the days and weeks following the simulation, they will reflect on and process these experience so that they may improve their performance as team members in the future.

A note about debriefing: it can be a difficult task to debrief a group of physicians and nurses who have just completed a simulated scenario. As stated earlier, team training simulations are high-stakes endeavors for the participants. Even though they are not receiving an evaluation, most health care providers who go through simulations have high expectations of themselves and are especially motivated to do well. Because the scenarios can be very realistic, participants often think that it could have been real. Because of this they may be disappointed in themselves if their performance is less than perfect. Identifying and accepting errors is part of the debriefing process. However, this may be very difficult for the debriefer who is tasked with debriefing health care providers who have self-expectations of perfection. Rudolph and colleagues[27] describe an excellent technique in briefing with good judgment.

Faculty Development

Planning, implementing, running, and especially debriefing a simulation all require skills and practice. These skills are specialized. Acquiring them is necessary before debriefing or having a leadership role in a simulation course. Probably the most effective way to start doing simulation is to take an introductory course in simulation instruction. The best way to obtain information on such a course is to contact a local simulation center or one of the simulation societies, such as the Society for Simulation in Healthcare or the International Pediatric Simulation Society.

Simulation-Based Teamwork Training in Otolaryngology

Improving teamwork in the OR is one of the ways to significantly reduce intraoperative and postoperative morbidity. Otolaryngologists, like other surgical specialists, are prone to increased risks in surgery secondary to poor teamwork performance. No matter where they practice, otolaryngologists may be called on to manage difficult airway situations. These potentially life-threatening circumstances are rare and occur acutely. Managing them well requires a well-prepared team that is both familiar with the procedures and equipment and is able to anticipate the possible complications. The nature of simulation-based team training makes it indispensable in preparing for these types of emergency cases (recall the 2-minute drills mentioned earlier).

Team training in otolaryngology is in its infancy. There are currently few otolaryngology programs in the country that have developed an otolaryngology-specific team training course. Despite this there are opportunities to participate in CRM training through anesthesia clinicians, who often have extensive simulation programs. Because they frequently deal with airway issues, anesthesiologists may welcome input from an otolaryngology colleague. Consider the possibility of joining them to either participate in a course or help plan a simulation-based course together.

Efficacy of Simulation

Just as the airline industry changed its culture and improved its safety record, it is imperative that health care does the same. As stated earlier, part of the underlying issue with the culture of health care is the isolated manner by which health care providers are educated. This will continue to have a deleterious effect on how multidisciplinary teams work together. Simulation-based team training is still not commonly used in many places. Teamwork training among health care providers is becoming more widespread. However, the number of practitioners in the health care systems is large so the proportion of caregivers who have consistently received simulation-based teamwork training remains small. However, there remains the question of how efficacious simulation-based learning is in improving teamwork and patient outcomes. It is clear that simulation improves people's ability to perform during subsequent simulations. There are several studies that suggest that simulation improves teamwork. Wayne and colleagues[28] showed that simulation-based training improves performance during actual cardiac resuscitations. Weller and colleagues[29] showed that simulation improves the Behavioral Marker Risk Index (BMRI), a teamwork and communication measurement tool, in general surgery teams compared with presimulation measures.

Improved attitudes toward teamwork in the OR have correlated with decreased postoperative mortality.[30] Steinemann and colleagues[31] showed that in situ simulation-based team training in trauma units has brought about improvement in teamwork scores compared with presimulation levels. More importantly, there was an improvement in the speed and completeness of the resuscitations of patients after the implementation of simulation-based training.[31] Mazzocco and colleagues and Haynes and Coleagues[16,30] showed that, in the OR, surgical performance and chance of mortality are strongly influence by the level of teamwork between OR personnel. In an extensive meta-analysis of simulation-based education articles, Cook and colleagues[32] showed that simulation-based training was associated with improved patient outcomes compared with no training. Woodward and colleagues,[33] in a review evaluating interventions to reduce medical errors, stated that medical simulation to improve team training should be part of a "hierarchy of error-reduction strategies." Many studies like these have shown that simulation-based team training improves teamwork and the attitudes of individuals toward teamwork. Such measures correlate with good patient outcomes. However, to date it has been difficult to prove that team training has a direct positive effect on patient safety.

SUMMARY

There continues to be an epidemic of health care errors. Because they occur in isolation and are usually beyond public scrutiny, their occurrence is largely underestimated by caregivers, patients and the general public. The most common causes of these errors are secondary to poor communication and team performance. Errors by individuals will always occur. Health care needs to rely on high-functioning teams to identify those errors and prevent them from causing patient harm. To do so, medicine needs to change the organizational, educational and cultural portions of its culture that impede formation of high-performance health care teams. Simulation-based team training is an educational tool that has brought about culture change and safety improvements in aviation and other high-stakes industries. At present, efforts are being made to develop multidisciplinary medical simulation courses to teach teamwork and safety culture within the OR. Such courses are considered high-fidelity simulation and are at a SimZone level of 4. These courses can take place in either a simulator center or in situ at the point of care. Outlined earlier in this article are some the challenges in scheduling, designing, running, and debriefing such a course.

Studies have shown that team training using medical simulation has the capability to change medical culture and enable health care teams to perform better. Research is ongoing to connect the use of simulation-based team training with improved patient outcomes. With more widespread use of medical simulation in the future, it is anticipated that such a connection will be established.

Otolaryngologists ordinarily have the potential of being involved in emergency management of the airway while in the operating room. Optimization of such emergencies is attained with good interdisciplinary teamwork. Otolaryngology is beginning to utilize medical simulation to improve team training by learning and practicing CRM principles. Future expansion of the role of medical simulation in otolaryngology will likely serve to enhance teamwork and improve patient safety.

REFERENCES

1. Gaba DM, DeAnda A. A comprehensive anesthesia simulation environment: recreating the operating room for research and training. Anesthesiology 1988; 69(3):387–94.

2. Kohn LT, Corrigan JM, and Donaldson MS, Editors; Committee on Quality of Health Care in America, Institute of Medicine: To Err Is Human: Building a Safer Health System. Washington, DC: National Academy Press. 1999.
3. Starfield B. Deficiencies in US medical care. JAMA 2000;284(17):2184–5.
4. James JT. A new, evidence-based estimate of patient harms associated with hospital care. J Patient Saf 2013;9(3):122–8.
5. Gawande AA, Thomas EJ, Zinner MJ, et al. The incidence and nature of surgical adverse events in Colorado and Utah in 1992. Surgery 1999;126(1):66–75.
6. Leape LL, Brennan TA, Laird N, et al. The nature of adverse events in hospitalized patients. Results of the Harvard Medical Practice Study II. N Engl J Med 1991; 324(6):377–84.
7. Sentinel event alert issue 30–July 21, 2004. Preventing infant death and injury during delivery. Adv Neonatal Care 2004;4(4):180–1.
8. Singh H, Thomas EJ, Petersen LA, et al. Medical errors involving trainees: a study of closed malpractice claims from 5 insurers. Arch Intern Med 2007;167(19): 2030–6.
9. Lingard L. Communication failures in the operating room: an observational classification of recurrent types and effects. Qual Saf Health Care 2004;13(5):330–4.
10. Christian CK, Gustafson ML, Roth EM, et al. A prospective study of patient safety in the operating room. Surgery 2006;139(2):159–73.
11. Landrigan CP, Parry GJ, Bones CB, et al. Temporal trends in rates of patient harm resulting from medical care. N Engl J Med 2010;363(22):2124–34.
12. Landgren R, Alawadi Z, Douma C, et al. Barriers of pediatric residents to speaking up about patient safety. Hosp Pediatr 2016;6(12):738–43.
13. Sexton JB, Thomas EJ, Helmreich RL. Error, stress, and teamwork in medicine and aviation: cross sectional surveys. BMJ 2000;320(7237):745–9.
14. Weller J, Boyd M, Cumin D. Teams, tribes and patient safety: overcoming barriers to effective teamwork in healthcare. Postgrad Med J 2014;90(1061):149–54.
15. Hudson B. Interprofessionality in health and social care: the Achilles' heel of partnership? J Interprof Care 2009;16(1):7–17.
16. Mazzocco K, Petitti DB, Fong KT, et al. Surgical team behaviors and patient outcomes. Am J Surg 2009;197(5):678–85.
17. Nagpal K, Vats A, Ahmed K, et al. An evaluation of information transfer through the continuum of surgical care: a feasibility study. Ann Surg 2010;252(2):402–7.
18. Volk MS, Ward J, Irias N, et al. Using medical simulation to teach crisis resource management and decision-making skills to otolaryngology housestaff. Otolaryngol Head Neck Surg 2011;145(1):35–42.
19. Brannick MT, Salas E, Prince C. Team performance assessment and measurement: theory, methods, and applications. Series in applied psychology. Mahwah (NJ): Lawrence Erlbaum Associates; 1997. p. 3–16.
20. Aviation SMo. Joint report: collision aeronaves Boeing 747 KLM Boeing 747 PANAM. 1978.
21. National Transportation Safety Board, editor. report number NTSB-AAR-73-14. Aircraft accident report, Eastern Airlines, Inc, L1011, N310EA Miami, FL 1972.
22. National Transportation Safety Board, editor. Report number NTSB-AAR-70-7. Aircraft accident report, United Airlines, Inc, McDonnell-Douglas, DC-8-81, M8082U Portland, OR 1978.
23. Schulz K. Being wrong: adventures in the margin of error. 1st edition. New York: Ecco; 2010.
24. Roussin CJ, Weinstock P. SimZones: an organizational innovation for simulation programs and centers. Acad Med 2017;92(8):1114–20.

25. Weinstock PH, Kappus LJ, Garden A, et al. Simulation at the point of care: reduced-cost, in situ training via a mobile cart. Pediatr Crit Care Med 2009; 10(2):176–81.

26. Kolb DA. Experiential learning: experience as the source of learning and development. Englewood Cliffs (NJ): Prentice-Hall; 1984.

27. Rudolph JW, Simon R, Rivard P, et al. Debriefing with good judgment: combining rigorous feedback with genuine inquiry. Anesthesiol Clin 2007;25(2):361–76.

28. Wayne DB, Didwania A, Feinglass J, et al. Simulation-based education improves quality of care during cardiac arrest team responses at an academic teaching hospital: a case-control study. Chest 2008;133(1):56–61.

29. Weller J, Cumin D, Torrie J, et al. Multidisciplinary operating room simulation-based team training to reduce treatment errors: a feasibility study in New Zealand hospitals. N Z Med J 2015;128(1418):40–51.

30. Haynes AB, Weiser TG, Berry WR, et al. Changes in safety attitude and relationship to decreased postoperative morbidity and mortality following implementation of a checklist-based surgical safety intervention. BMJ Qual Saf 2011;20(1): 102–7.

31. Steinemann S, Berg B, Skinner A, et al. In situ, multidisciplinary, simulation-based teamwork training improves early trauma care. J Surg Educ 2011;68(6):472–7.

32. Cook DA, Hatala R, Brydges R, et al. Technology-enhanced simulation for health professions education: a systematic review and meta-analysis. JAMA 2011; 306(9):978–88.

33. Woodward HI, Mytton OT, Lemer C, et al. What have we learned about interventions to reduce medical errors? Annu Rev Public Health 2010;31:479–97, 471 p following 497.

Facilitation and Debriefing in Simulation Education

Sarah N. Bowe, MD[a],*, Kaalan Johnson, MD[b], Liana Puscas, MD, MHS, MA[c]

KEYWORDS

- Otolaryngology • Simulation • Education • Facilitation • Feedback • Debriefing

KEY POINTS

- Facilitation requires enumeration of educational goals, a realistically designed and executed scenario, and clear articulation of the ground rules of the scenario.
- Structured debriefing is essential to accomplish the educational goals of the simulation.
- Debriefing focused on specific thought processes and actions helps participants to identify knowledge and communication gaps and analyze the outcome of those thoughts and actions.
- The general structure of most debriefing sessions focuses on participant reactions, followed by analysis, and ending with a discussion of lessons learned.
- The 2 leading debriefing models include the Structured and Supported Debriefing Model and the Debriefing with Good Judgment Model.

The goal of this article was to equip those interested in simulation with 2 essential tools for success: facilitation of and debriefing after a simulated scenario. As simulation is still an emerging area in otolaryngology education, many faculty and residents may not be familiar with the technical aspects of facilitating simulation and leading a good debriefing session. In this article, we explain the theoretic foundations of facilitation and debriefing, enumerate key principles of facilitation and debriefing, and describe 2 different, common approaches to debriefing. After reading this article, one should be able to recall the basic principles of facilitating a simulated scenario and debriefing session and use these techniques to develop a scenario and provide feedback after a simulation experience.

None of the authors have any commercial or financial conflicts of interest. There were no funding sources for this article.

[a] Department of Otolaryngology–Head and Neck Surgery, Massachusetts Eye and Ear, 243 Charles Street, Boston, MA 02114, USA; [b] Division of Otolaryngology, Head and Neck Surgery, Seattle Children's Hospital, 4800 Sand Point Way Northeast, Seattle, WA 98105, USA; [c] Division of Head and Neck Surgery and Communication Sciences, Duke University Medical Center Box 3805, Durham, NC 27710, USA
* Corresponding author.
E-mail address: Sarah_Bowe@meei.harvard.edu

Otolaryngol Clin N Am 50 (2017) 989–1001
http://dx.doi.org/10.1016/j.otc.2017.05.009
0030-6665/17/Published by Elsevier Inc.

THEORETIC FOUNDATION OF FACILITATION AND DEBRIEFING
Facilitation

Successful simulation begins with appropriate facilitation. By definition, a simulated experience is an engineered situation. The flow of the scenario and the degree to which the objectives of the simulation are achieved are in large measure the result of the skill of the facilitator(s). There are several fundamental principles and techniques that underlie effective facilitation, and these have been simplified for the purposes of this discussion.[1,2]

Facilitation encompasses 3 aspects, which may be categorized along a chronologic spectrum: prescenario, intrascenario, and postscenario.

1. Prescenario:
   a. Enumerate the educational objectives. The facilitator(s) must know the primary and secondary goals of the scenario. The decision to share the objectives with the participants will be up to the choice of the instructor. Objectives, however, do not need to be shared with the participants (eg, the goal of an airway scenario might be to perform a cricothyrotomy), as part of the educational process can be allowing the learners to come to that conclusion themselves.
   b. Create as realistic a simulation as possible, which helps participants to immerse themselves in the situation.
   c. Clearly articulate the ground rules of the scenario. Explain the setting, the roles of the individual participants, and the need for them to suspend reality to achieve the goals of this artificial construct.
2. Intrascenario:
   a. Allow the scenario to progress without interruption. Even though the settings on the mannequin or scenario details may be manipulated to drive the participants toward the educational goals, one should not interfere with the decisions of the participants.
   b. Use confederates to help accomplish educational goals. Fellow facilitators who remain in character play key roles in the progression of the scenario and are valuable sources of observation and feedback.
   c. Adjust the "signal-to-noise ratio" to fit the training level of the participants. How much distraction (noise), if any, is incorporated into the scenario and how many additional cues (signal) are needed, if any, to bring the participants through the educational objectives?
3. Postscenario. The postscenario aspect of debriefing is discussed in further detail throughout the remainder of the article.

Debriefing

Debriefing is related to the adult learning principle of experiential learning as described by Malcolm Knowles. Adults often learn best by undergoing new experiences and augmenting learning acquired from prior ones. Case studies, role-playing, simulation, and reflection on decisions and outcomes provide the framework of learning through experience.[3] This last aspect of consideration of decisions and actions is the focus of debriefing. Most otolaryngologists have engaged in this activity without having given it a formal name: discussing a bad outcome or a near miss in Morbidity and Mortality Conference, critiquing a resident's operative or clinic performance, performing a root cause analysis, and so forth. In these situations, questions such as "What was the thought process behind that decision?" or "What could you/I have done differently?" are asked, and participants learn from this process.

Formal debriefing is an intentional discussion that helps "participants of simulation gain a clear understanding of their performance during the session."[4] However, the principles of simulation debriefing, such as feedback from the facilitator, verbalizing of impressions, and reviewing actions and perceptions, can be applied to any situation in which discussion of actions after the fact is held. Debriefing after simulation, or after a planned intervention/educational session, though, has the distinct advantage of being able to integrate the educational objectives of the activity into the debriefing process, thus ensuring that those goals are met.

Debriefing is one of the most important components that contributes to the effectiveness of simulation-based learning, so it is important to understand its underpinnings.[5–7] David Kolb[8] clearly articulated the importance of reflection and analysis in his development of Experiential Learning Theory. Donald Schön[9] focused on professionals and their capacity to self-reflect on their actions, which results in a process of continuing learning and improvement. K. Anders Ericsson[10,11] has written persuasively that repetition and feedback are essential for performance improvement.

Paul Phrampus and John O'Donnell[4] have elegantly distilled the best practices of debriefing and these are further simplified below.

- The gap in time between performance and debriefing should be as short as possible.
- Performance and perception gaps should be identified and addressed.
- A "social" aspect must be considered to enhance learner comfort and participation.
- Participants must engage in self-reflection.
- Instructors must have facilitation and debriefing skills.
- Debriefing cannot be comprehensive and should focus on only a few aspects/educational goals of an activity (ie, faculty/facilitators cannot address all possible teaching points but instead must ensure that a few key points are made).
- Debriefing requires structure to achieve its objectives; that is, the exclusive use of broad, open-ended questions, such as "What happened?" may not achieve the educational aims as well as asking "What was your thought process when you first saw the patient?"

As can be seen, the role of the faculty/facilitator is key to a successful debriefing session.[4] The faculty must establish an engaging and supportive context for teaching so that participants can honestly assess their performance, and, together, faculty and learners can identify gaps and ways to improve. Successful faculty will use various communication techniques to ensure that debriefing results in a fruitful discussion. Faculty must engage in active listening and remain closely attuned to the nonverbal cues provided by the participants. It is beneficial to restate participant comments and summarize these to improve clarity for everyone in the group. Asking probing questions to elicit participant thought processes helps learners correlate thoughts with actions and provides essential opportunities to identify and correct performance gaps (or reinforce appropriate decisions). Linking the simulation scenario with real-world situations gets to the heart of successful simulation because it allows participants to clearly see the relevance of what they are learning. Finally, a good facilitator will appropriately redirect the discussion so that essential teaching points are covered while also capitalizing on what learners identified as new knowledge.

FEEDBACK: THE HEART OF DEBRIEFING

Feedback is considered the single most important feature of simulation-based education toward the goal of effective learning.[12] Van de Ridder and colleagues[13] recently operationalized the definition of feedback in clinical education as "specific information about the comparison between a trainee's observed performance and a standard, given with the intent to improve the trainee's performance." Depending on the type of educational activity, feedback may be brief and simple or detailed and complex. To attain the most effective feedback, Motola and colleagues[14] recommend focusing on the 3 Ps of feedback: planning, prebriefing, and providing feedback/debriefing.

Planning

The planning stage brings the focus back to the learning objectives that were identified during scenario development. Learning objectives have been defined as "2 to 3 observable accomplishments of learners following a simulation session."[15] Therefore, clear objectives help to focus the facilitator's observations during the scenario so that specific behavioral examples can be provided later in the feedback process. This also provides the opportunity for the educator to develop short didactic "lecturettes" to describe evidence-based guidelines or best practices related to a given learning objective.[15]

During a simulation activity, it is equally important for the instructor to examine learner-generated or "emergent" objectives.[16] These objectives are not predetermined, but arise during the simulation, such as an obvious knowledge gap or systems issue that should not be overlooked. In most cases, not all objectives can be discussed and the educator must determine which objectives will take precedence for that particular feedback session.

Prebrief

The main purpose of the prebrief is to create a psychologically safe context for learning, which allows active engagement despite potential threats to professional and social identity.[17] Rudolph and colleagues[17] recognize 4 discrete activities that can foster psychological safety within the simulation environment. First, the facilitator should introduce himself or herself, including credentials and relevant experience, and then encourage all simulation participants to do the same. At the same time, it can be beneficial for faculty to propose a personal goal, thus modeling an environment in which it is safe to share feelings and emotions. In addition, clarity about the learning objectives, simulator properties, scenario design, and type of assessment (ie, formative vs summative) can be provided. Second, the instructor should establish the "fiction contract," acknowledging the limitations inherent within the simulation environment (eg, mannequin's skin color does not change), stating his or her efforts to make the scenario as real as possible, and seeking a commitment from the participants to perform as if they would in a real-life situation. Third, attending to logistical detail (eg, session timing, breaks, pager handling) helps participants focus more completely on the simulation exercise. Finally, facilitators should convey respect and interest in the learner's perspective, which can lead to a deeper understanding of his or her thoughts and emotions that influence behavior.[17]

Providing Feedback/Debriefing

Simulation educational methods are diverse, ranging from partial task training with students to complicated, interdisciplinary team training with working professionals. Various debriefing models have emerged based on a multitude of factors, including method of instruction, learner experience, amount of time available for simulation exercise, equipment capability, and physical facilities (eg, audiovisual equipment, observation areas, debriefing rooms).[4] Furthermore, the level of expertise and number of instructors also will determine how debriefing is performed. A detailed description of every model is beyond the scope of this work. The general structure of most debriefing sessions focuses on participant reactions, followed by analysis, and ending with a discussion of lessons learned. **Box 1** provides a general summary of common debriefing models. Two leading debriefing models are presented in further detail as follows.

Box 1
Models of the debriefing process

Thatcher and Robinson[21]

1. Identifying the impact of the experience
2. Identifying and considering the processes that developed
3. Clarifying the facts, concepts, and principles
4. Identifying the ways in which emotion was involved
5. Identifying the different views that each of the participants formed

Lederman[22]

1. Introduction to systematic reflection and analysis
2. Intensification and personalization of the analysis of the experience
3. Generalization and application of the experience

Petranek[23]

1. Events
2. Emotions
3. Empathy
4. Explanations and analysis
5. Everyday applicability
6. Employment of information
7. Evaluation

Owen and Follows[24] (GREAT)

1. Guidelines
2. Recommendations
3. Events
4. Analysis
5. Transfer of knowledge to clinical practice

Rudolph et al[25] (Debriefing with Good Judgment)

1. Reactions
2. Analysis
3. Summary

O'Donnell et al[26] (Structured and Supported Debriefing)

1. Gather
2. Analyze
3. Summarize

Structured and Supported Debriefing Model

The Winter Institute for Simulation Education and Research (WISER) at the University of Pittsburgh is a high-volume, multidisciplinary simulation center with a mission to conduct training programs and research using simulation-based education. In 2009, WISER collaborated with the American Heart Association to develop a model for debriefing advanced cardiac life support and pediatric advanced life support scenarios.[18] From this effort, the Structured and Supported Debriefing model was developed. The Structured component is derived from 3 specific debriefing phases with focused goals, actions, and time-allocation estimates. The Supported component arises from the creation of an environment with interpersonal support, as well as the use of protocols and best evidence to support the debriefing process.[18]

The acronym for the Structured portion of this model is GAS, standing for gather, analyze, and summarize, which provides an organized approach to guide the debriefing session.[4] As a reminder, throughout each of the debriefing phases, the facilitator must remain cognizant of the initial learning objectives for which the simulation was designed.

Gather The goals of this phase are to gather information that will be used to facilitate the later phases. At the beginning of the phase, participants are invited to share their thoughts and feelings about the session. This is the initial chance to decompress from the simulation activity. The use of open-ended questions, such as "What are your thoughts?" or "How did that make you feel?" provides an opportunity for open dialogue and may begin to reveal those topics most pertinent to the participants.

In addition, the facilitator can begin to identify perception versus performance gaps.[4] Perception gaps refer to the dissonance between the participants' perception of their performance compared with those by the facilitator. To recall, feedback is intended to provide "specific information about the comparison between a trainee's observed performance and a standard, given with the intent to improve the trainee's performance."[13] The perception gap must be considered primarily as the ability to perceive and self-assess performance that will frame the remaining portions of the debriefing. In particular, it is critical to identify those times in which there are wide perception gaps, in which there is complete discordance between the perceptions of the participants and those of the facilitator.[4] When there is a wide perception gap, the remainder of the gather phase must be directed at understanding the participants' thoughts or feelings to fully understand their perceptions and work to close the perception gap throughout the remaining phases of debriefing.

In contrast, when there is a narrow perception gap, and the learners and facilitators are in agreement with the simulation performance, then the remainder of the gather phase can be used to clarify information that can be used to close a performance gap. Performance gaps are defined as the gap between desired and actual performance. In this situation, the facilitator may use probing questions to identify the rationale (eg, feelings, beliefs, assumptions, knowledge base) that led to the actions or behaviors that were observed during the simulation. Once the instructor has identified sufficient information to address either perception or performance gaps throughout the remainder of the debriefing, there is a transition to the analyze phase. In total, the gather phase should take approximately 25% of the total debriefing time.[4]

Analyze The analyze phase generally begins with a brief synopsis of the appropriate decision pathway of the scenario. In general, it is beneficial for the facilitator to have a 1-sentence or 2-sentence summary of the intended course of action that can be provided succinctly in a nonjudgmental manner. This also can provide a useful segue to introduce the first topic to be examined in the analyze phase. In most cases, the 2 or 3 learning objectives provide the focus for topics to be discussed during the analyze phase. The skilled instructor, however, must also remain vigilant during the gather phase for any "emergent" objectives that must not be overlooked.[16] Therefore, the facilitator must continuously direct and redirect the conversation to achieve the session's intended objectives.

The goal of the analyze phase is to encourage reflection on behalf of the participants to promote self-discovery.[4] The focus of this self-reflection will depend on the skill level of the participants. The "conscious competence" learning model can help to guide the conversation during the analyze phase[9] (**Fig. 1**). Participants who have been identified to have a perception gap are generally in the beginning "unconscious incompetence" stage of learning. Their inability to recognize the deficit in their performance serves as the driver for the perception gap. As a result, questions during the analyze phase would ideally encourage the participants to recognize their "incompetence," therefore moving them toward the second stage of "conscious incompetence." When a perception gap exists, simply enlightening the learners to the presence of a wide perception gap, and closing this gap, may be the goal for a given simulation session.

On the other hand, during the gather phase, the facilitator may have identified a narrow perception gap, such that the views of the learner and instructor are in alignment. When this occurs, the focus of the analyze phase can be directed at the closure of performance gaps or possibly improvement on good performance. The "conscious competence" model also can be informative in this setting. When both the facilitator and learner have identified poor performance, the learner is exhibiting "conscious incompetence." The learner is able to recognize the deficit in his or her thinking or skills and reflect on these deficits with the help of the facilitator. This can be an ideal time to incorporate cognitive aids (eg, management algorithms) and provide short didactic "lecturettes" or skills training.[4] This can provide the participant with the added skill or knowledge to bring him or her to "conscious competence." At this point, the participant possess the prerequisite information and ability, but still must concentrate and focus to perform well.[9]

In some cases, the narrow performance gap, where the learner and facilitator have both identified a strong performance, may be the hardest scenario to debrief. In this case, the instructor is potentially dealing with participants with "conscious competence" with little cognitive or technical performance gaps. Or, the instructor may be dealing with participants who even have "unconscious competence," having so much experience that the activity has become "second nature."[19] In these situations, the intended learning objectives were achieved. Thus, the facilitator must adapt, ideally drawing from the information obtained during the gather phase. For example, there may be opportunities to identify interpersonal communication or systems-based issues that occurred during the simulation. Another potential option would

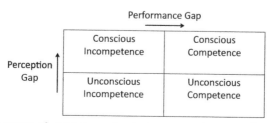

Fig. 1. Advancing stages of competence by closing perception or performance gaps.

be to engage participants in describing any similar real-life experiences in which there might have been a poor outcome and reflect on differences between the two. Perhaps, a real-life encounter provided the learning opportunity that allowed success to occur during the simulation and this can be shared with other participants.

Overall, the analyze phase draws from the information obtained during the gather phase and guides participants to reflect and advance along the competence continuum. In total, the analyze phase should take approximately 50% of the total debriefing time.[4] At this point, there is a transition to the final summarize phase.

Summarize The goal of the summarize phase is to ensure a clear understanding of the most important take-away points.[4] In fact, it is often recommended that there is a clear transition made by the facilitator. For example, "Ok, I think we've had a great discussion on a number of topics, let's talk about the main points we are going to take away from this session." In many cases, the main take-away points will reflect back on the initial learning objectives, but there may have been "emergent" objectives that took precedence during the session and should be included in the take-home points.

In the Structured and Supported Debriefing model, the summarize phase is organized around a plus-delta technique.[4] The plus-delta is a model focused on effective actions or behaviors (+) and actions or behaviors that could undergo improvement (Δ). During the summarize phase, participants would be asked to provide 2 positive aspects of performance and 2 areas they would change the next time they encountered a similar scenario. The instructor also has the option to perform a final summary, providing an overall plus-delta to complete the summarize phase, which should take the remaining 25% of the total debriefing time.[4]

Debriefing with Good Judgment Model

Debriefing after an educational experience has a powerful ability to uncover a participant's personal frame of reference and allow a reorganization and expansion of the educational framework. An alternative approach to simulation education and debriefing capitalizing on this concept has been proposed by the Center for Medical Simulation in Cambridge, Massachusetts, and taught to thousands of simulation educators through their courses, called "Debriefing with Good Judgment."[15] This is characterized by 4 key principles: (1) defining learning objectives clearly before the simulation session, (2) setting expectations clearly for the session, (3) approaching learners with true curiosity and feedback while avoiding the urge to "fix" learners, and (4) organizing the debriefing session into 3 phases: reactions, analysis, and summary (using the advocacy/inquiry technique).

Reactions The reactions phase of the debriefing is the opportunity to clear the air, relax, and breathe after an often emotionally charged, generally stressful, and always new and stretching educational experience. Very similar to the "Gather" phase described previously, this phase begins with questions such as "How did that feel?" and allows faculty to hear initial reactions, validate emotional responses, and make note of potential learner-generated goals for the debriefing session. This should be an opportunity to clarify any critical facts of the scenario; for example, "this scenario involved a pneumothorax that progressed into tension physiology," or "the nurse in this scenario was new on this floor and had never been oriented to the process for calling the code team." Giving the punchline at this stage in the debriefing allows learners to begin the work of analyzing their frame of reference during the scenario and optimizing their learning potential from the exercise. The reactions phase is composed of feelings and facts.

Analysis The analysis phase allows the facilitator and learners to work together to observe gaps between desired and actual performance, investigate the basis for and provide feedback on these gaps, and work toward closing these gaps through discussion and didactics as appropriate. Performance gaps will not be uniform among a group of learners and will not be perceived equally by each learner. The analysis phase allows the opportunity to come to unity on the content and extent of these gaps so that they can be effectively addressed for each learner.

A nonjudgmental debriefing technique that is sometimes used during the analysis phase is a concept called the "Debriefing Molecule," which is composed of Curiosity as the core atom, surrounded by equal parts of Advocacy and Inquiry[20] (**Fig. 2**). This construct encourages the facilitator to always maintain at the core the deep desire to understand the learner's frame of reference with true curiosity, which sets the stage for communicating a desire to help the learner change and progress in learning and skill. Then, specific questions are posed during the analysis to advocate for the cognitive dissonance experienced by the facilitator (Advocacy), such as "I observed…" or "I am concerned/pleased that…" followed by concrete examples of what the facilitator had observed of actions that were pertinent to a learning objective during the scenario and how this may illustrate a performance gap. This is followed by an open-ended question (Inquiry) to understand the learner's perspective or frame of reference, such as "What was on your mind at that time?" or "How did you see that?"

Summary The summary phase is the opportunity for the facilitator to allow learners to share insights as they complete their analysis of past and future performance and prepare to "take home" the main points that they hope to use when the clinical scenario presents itself again. This is generally led by the learners unless important learning objectives are omitted and may be shared by the facilitators. It allows the learners to fully process and summarize what they plan to retain from this experience, and ideally

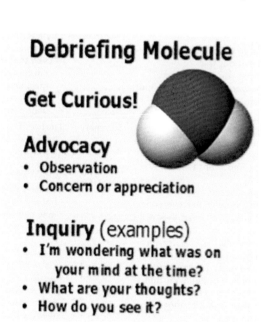

Debriefing Molecule

Get Curious!

Advocacy
- Observation
- Concern or appreciation

Inquiry (examples)
- I'm wondering what was on your mind at the time?
- What are your thoughts?
- How do you see it?

Fig. 2. Visual summary of advocacy/inquiry approach to debriefing. (*Courtesy of* Center for Medical Simulation, Boston, MA. www.harvardmedsim.org.)

implement a plan for operationalizing this knowledge when it is required in the clinical setting[15].

SUMMARY

Facilitation and debriefing of a simulation session is a challenging and critical skill to develop when embarking on simulation education. The ability of a facilitator to create a welcoming learning environment in which learners are able to fully participate in a simulation scenario; open up about their thoughts, actions, and frame of reference during a debriefing; and fully assimilate the learning objectives of the

Table 1
Comparison of the structured and supported debriefing model and the debriefing with good judgment model

Structured and Supported Debriefing		Debriefing with Good Judgment	
Phase	Sample Questions/Language	Phase	Sample Questions/Language
Gather	"What are you thinking?" "What are your thoughts?" "How did that make you feel?"	Reactions	Feelings "How did that feel?" "What are your initial thoughts?" "What are your immediate reactions?"
Analyze	"Before we delve deeper, I'd like to review the intended management for this scenario." "Before we get started, I'd like to go over the appropriate steps for managing this patient." "I noticed that you.... Tell me more about that." "How did you feel when....?" "What were you thinking about when....?"	Analysis	Facts "First, I'd like to take a few minutes to present the facts of the case." "Before we move on, I'd like to review the case so that everyone is on the same page." Advocacy/Inquiry "I saw that you waited until.... I'm concerned that the delay may have resulted in.... I'm wondering what was on your mind at that time?"
Summarize	"Thank you all for your comments. I think we've had a great discussion. Let's consider some important take-away points." "We've covered a number of topics, now I'd like everyone to think about what they want to take away from this experience." "Let's go around the room and I'd like everyone to identify one action or behavior that went well and one action or behavior that if changed would lead to better performance."	Summary	"I noticed that you.... I think that helped others to recognize.... I'm wondering what you were thinking at then." "When the patient was...., I noticed that....was happening. I think that this may have caused.... How do you see it?" "Thank you for your participation. Our debriefing session is coming to a close. I'd like to invite each of you to share your thoughts on what went well, as well as what you might hope to change or improve in the future."

simulation session into actionable items of change in their clinical practice is absolutely paramount to the success of a simulation education event. Clearly enumerating educational objectives for simulation education experiences, facilitating to match participant experience level to simulation content, and using appropriate techniques for debriefing, such as "Structured and Supported Debriefing (GAS),"[4] "Debriefing with Good Judgment (RAS),"[15] and the advocacy/inquiry method[20] of analyzing participants' actions can make an enormous difference in the ability of participants to leave with actionable learning items from a simulation education session. **Table 1** provides a final summary of the primary debriefing techniques discussed previously. **Table 2** provides a list of organizations that provide focused opportunities for faculty and professional development specifically within health care simulation. We hope after completing this article that the reader will feel more fully equipped to successfully facilitate and debrief any simulation experience that is needed by their learners.

Table 2
List of organizations that offer training for health care simulation educators

Organization	Summary of Training
University of Pittsburgh Peter M. Winter Institute for Simulation, Education, and Research (WISER) (http://www.wiser.pitt.edu/)	Series of course offerings including an introduction to the fundamental skills and abilities for delivering simulation-based health care education (partner course to GCRME), best practices in simulation center design, and simulation operations specialist training
Center for Medical Simulation (https://harvardmedsim.org/)	Variety of programs for simulation leaders, educators, and researchers including debriefing skills, comprehensive experiential simulation education workshops, and interprofessional team-based training options
Mayo Clinic Multidisciplinary Simulation Centers (http://www.mayo.edu/multidisciplinary-simulation-center)	Faculty development workshops focused on course design and concepts and debriefing strategies through an interactive experience
University of Miami Michael S. Gordon Center for Research in Medical Education (GCRME) (http://www.crme.med.miami.edu/medical_education_teaching_programs.php)	Coursework focused on an introduction to the fundamental skills and abilities for delivering simulation-based health care education (partner course to WISER), as well as mannequin operations and programming
University of Washington Center for Health Sciences Interprofessional Education, Research, and Practice (http://collaborate.uw.edu/faculty-development/teaching-with-simulation/teaching-with-simulation.html-0)	Eight free, self-paced, Web-based modules including introduction to clinical simulation, pedagogical approaches to guide teaching, designing and writing a scenario, briefing and debriefing techniques, appropriate assessment using educational outcomes, enhancing realism, and preparing interprofessional simulation sessions

This list provides a representative sample of programs, but is not exhaustive. No endorsement of any particular program is implied.

REFERENCES

1. Franklin AE, Boese T, Gloe D, et al. Standards of best practice: simulation standard IV: facilitation. Clin Simul Nurs 2013;9:S19–21.
2. DeMaria S Jr, Levine AI. The use of stress to enrich the simulated environment. In: Levine AI, DeMaria S Jr, Schwartz AD, et al, editors. The comprehensive textbook of healthcare simulation. New York: Springer; 2013. p. 65–72.
3. Andragogy (Malcolm Knowles) (2015). Available at: http://www.instructionaldesign.org/theories.andragogy.html. Accessed November 5, 2016.
4. Phrampus PE, O'Donnell JM. Debriefing using a structured and supported approach. In: Levine AI, DeMaria S Jr, Schwartz AD, et al, editors. The comprehensive textbook of healthcare simulation. New York: Springer; 2013. p. 73–84.
5. Cantrell MA. The importance of debriefing in clinical simulations. Clin Simul Nurs 2008;4(2):e19–23.
6. McDonnell LK, Jobe KK, Dismukes RK. Facilitating LOS debriefings: a training manual. NASAN technical memorandum 112192. Mountain View (CA): Ames Research Center; 1997.
7. McGaghie WC, Isssenberg SB, Petrusa ER, et al. A critical review of simulation-based medical education research: 2003-2009. Med Educ 2010;44(1):50–63.
8. Kolb D. Experiential learning: experience as the source of learning and development. Upper Saddle River (NJ): Prentice-Hall; 1984.
9. Schön D. Educating the reflective practitioner: toward a new design for teaching and learning in the professions. 1st edition. San Francisco (CA): Jossey-Bass; 1987.
10. Ericsson KA. Deliberate practice and the acquisition and maintenance of expert performance in medicine and related domains. Acad Med 2004;79(10 Suppl):S70–81.
11. Ericsson KA. Deliberate practice and acquisition of expert performance: a general overview. Acad Emerg Med 2008;15(11):988–94.
12. Issenberg SB, Mcgaghie WC, Petrusa ER, et al. Features and uses of high-fidelity medical simulations that lead to effective learning: a BEME systematic review. Med Teach 2005;27:10–28.
13. van de Ridder JMM, Stokking KM, McGaghie WC, et al. What is feedback in clinical education? Med Educ 2008;42:189–97.
14. Motola I, Devine LA, Chung HS, et al. Simulation in healthcare education: a best evidence practical guide. AMEE Guide No. 82. Med Teach 2013;35:e1511–30.
15. Szyld D, Rudolph JW. Debriefing with good judgment. In: Levine AI, DeMaria S Jr, Schwartz AD, et al, editors. The comprehensive textbook of healthcare simulation. New York: Springer; 2013. p. 85–93.
16. Fanning RM, Gaba DM. The role of debriefing in simulation-based learning. Simul Healthc 2007;2:115–25.
17. Rudolph JW, Raemer DB, Simon R. Establishing a safe container for learning in simulation: the role of the presimulation briefing. Simul Healthc 2014;9:339–49.
18. American Heart Association. Structured and Supported Debriefing (February 2015). Available at: http://www.onlineaha.org/system/scidea/courses/29/more_info/SSD_LEARN_MORE.pdf. Accessed November 5, 2016.
19. Adam L. Learning a new skill is easier said than done (November 2016). Available at: http://www.gordontraining.com/free-workplace-articles/learning-a-new-skill-is-easier-said-than-done/. Accessed November 6, 2016.
20. Rogers P.. In Great evidence in medical education summary (GEMeS). 2016. Available at: https://canadiem.org/caep-gemes-effectiveness-feedback-faculty-learners-often-challenged-faculty-factors/. Accessed November 6, 2016.

21. Thatcher DC, Robinson MJ. An introduction to games and simulations in education. Hants: Solent Simulations; 1985.

22. Lederman LC. Differences that make a difference: intercultural communication, simulation, and the debriefing process in diverse interaction. Presented at the Annual Conference of the International Simulation and Gaming Association. Kyoto, Japan, July 15–19, 1991.

23. Petranek C. Maturation in experiential learning: principles of simulation and gaming. Simul Gaming 1994;25:513–22.

24. Owen H, Follows V. GREAT simulation debriefing. Med Educ 2006;40:488–9.

25. Rudolph JW, Simon R, Dufresne RL, et al. There's no such thing as "nonjudgmental" debriefing: a theory and method for debriefing with good judgment. Simul Healthc 2006;1:49–55.

26. O'Donnell JM, Rodgers D, Lee W, et al. Structured and supported debriefing (interactive multimedia program). Dallas (TX): American Heart Association; 2009.

Boot Camps

Preparing for Residency

David H. Yeh, MD[a], Kevin Fung, MD[a],*, Sonya Malekzadeh, MD[b]

KEYWORDS

- Otolaryngology • Boot camp • Simulation • Education

KEY POINTS

- Simulation-based boot camps are intensive events in which residents actively practice their psychomotor, cognitive, and affective skills.
- Course content and structure are based on participant needs and adult learning principles that emphasize hands-on learning, directed practice, and debriefing.
- Boot camp implementation requires considerable support and resources.
- Regionalization of boot camps may alleviate infrastructure limitations.
- Outcomes studies confirm improvement of self-perceived knowledge, skills, and behaviors.

INTRODUCTION

During the course of medical school, students are trained as relatively undifferentiated general physicians with a broad understanding of medicine. Electives and subinternships hone a student's interests, knowledge, and skills in a particular specialty, but ultimately, the transition from clerkship to residency can be abrupt and stressful. The dramatic increase in direct patient care and clinical responsibility may exacerbate this anxiety, especially in students who feel ill-equipped or lack self-confidence in their abilities.[1] Although all graduating medical students pass standardized examinations before becoming resident physicians, there is undoubtedly some variability in the fund of knowledge and skills among graduating medical students.

The cumulative effect of these factors, along with the sudden changeover of experienced house staff replaced with new trainees, has been shown to adversely affect patient care and outcomes. Studies have demonstrated a clear spike in errors

The authors have no commercial or financial conflicts of interest. There were no funding sources for this article.

[a] Department of Otolaryngology–Head and Neck Surgery, London Health Sciences Center, Victoria Hospital, 800 Commissioners Road East, London, Ontario N6A 5W9, Canada; [b] Department of Otolaryngology–Head and Neck Surgery, MedStar Georgetown University Hospital, 3800 Reservoir Road, Northwest, Washington, DC 20007, USA
* Corresponding author.
E-mail address: Kevin.fung@lhsc.on.ca

associated with increased mortality when new physicians take on clinical responsibilities in July.[2,3] Proposed solutions center on the premise that not all trainees at a given level possess the same skills. The most compelling approach is the introduction of focused training to balance the disparities, preferably before the new role is assumed.

Simulation-based education, and introductory boot camps, in particular, may serve as the optimum bridge between medical school and residency, equipping novice residents with the necessary foundational knowledge, procedural, and communication skills before undertaking clinical responsibilities relevant for their specialty. This article aims to provide an overview of otolaryngology boot camps and the current evidence supporting simulation boot camps in residency training.

BOOT CAMP CONCEPT

Boot camps in medical education are loosely based on military boot camps: the premise of both are similar in that the emphasis is to provide basic training for a relatively undifferentiated new recruit with the opportunity to acquire and practice the requisite skills necessary to fulfill their responsibilities.

Other high-stakes industries face similar challenges in training their novices. In the aviation sector, for example, pilots devote a significant portion of their training to simulations that prepare them for time-sensitive, critical, and crisis-averting decisions.[4] Simulations maximize their experience so when faced with similarly critical real-life situations, they draw from their simulation training. Similarly, offering simulation-based medical education early in otolaryngology training allows novice residents the opportunity to practice diagnostic, management, and technical skills before meeting these challenges in real-life situations.

In recent years, with the increasing emphasis on patient safety and improved outcomes, there is growing sentiment that the traditional model of resident education needs further refinement.[5] Moreover, surgical residency programs are required to enforce duty-hour restriction, possibly limiting the trainee's exposure to rare but critical and life-threatening situations.[4] As a result, the traditional teaching mantra of "see one, do one, teach one" with real-life patients is being challenged. Simulation-based medical education and boot camps provide trainees with structured learning in an intensive and immersive environment allowing deliberate practice of skills and behaviors in the management of real-life scenarios. Other benefits include a distraction-free and nonthreatening environment in which learners receive immediate feedback All this can be achieved while minimizing patient risk and discomfort.[6–10] These interactive experiences can entail standardized patients, virtual reality simulators, task trainers, and human patient simulation.

Many specialties, including general surgery, vascular surgery, emergency medicine, and anesthesia use boot camps to transition trainees into their new role as residents.[2] In the United States, the Society of Neurological Surgeons hosts standardized and mandatory regional boot camps for all PGY-1 (postgraduate year) neurosurgery residents across the country.[11,12] Similarly, otolaryngology boot camps can be designed to introduce important principles of otolaryngology care to novice residents, including hands-on practice with a variety of exercises to develop the cognitive, communication, and procedural skills necessary for an otolaryngology residency.

INTENDED LEARNERS

Novice residents are expected to possess baseline skills at the onset of residency, largely because they are the first responders to most otolaryngology calls and consults. However, the reality remains that most new residents have limited exposure to common airway and bleeding emergencies and are likely unprepared in managing these scenarios. Currently, most otolaryngology boot camps are designed to onboard junior trainees embarking on their residency. These annual courses in the United States, Canada, and the United Kingdom are proliferating with similar objectives to meet the needs of their respective learners.[9,13–15]

Otolaryngology disorders are common in primary care and emergency room settings, representing 20% to 50% of complaints.[16] Primary care providers must be able to identify pathology, initiate the first steps of management, or even treat the condition. This is especially paramount in remote settings where otolaryngologists may not be available. The boot camp course at Western University in Canada has, in recent years, integrated learners from other specialties, such as rural emergency medicine. A knowledgeable and skilled emergency room physician, equipped to address otolaryngology emergencies in remote locations, has immeasurable benefits for patients and the health care system. Similarly, integrating anesthesiology residents into an acute airway management session during a boot camp would allow better communication and a mutual appreciation of each specialty's capabilities and limitations; these shared experiences could prove invaluable during a real-life airway emergency.

With the ongoing changes in the medical industry and emphasis on cost-efficient solutions to health care delivery, extended-care providers are taking on new and advanced responsibilities. Boot camps can provide physician assistants and nurse practitioners with the skills and tools to transition into their expanding role in health care. Multidisciplinary teams or interprofessional learners may benefit from an otolaryngology boot camp. Nurses and other allied health care providers, such as respiratory therapists, may be the first on the scene in otolaryngology emergencies; they will need to recognize, triage, and initiate management for these emergencies. Enhancing their knowledge and understanding of otolaryngology disorders and procedures can result in improvement of patient outcomes.

CURRICULUM DESIGN

Before developing a course curriculum, educators should conduct a formal assessment of the educational goals of the prospective learner or learner group. A needs assessment characterizes the difference between existing knowledge of the learner and the purpose of the learning encounter. This information can be obtained by directly querying the learners or the faculty about their perceptions of the educational needs, formally testing learners, or identifying specific requirements set by academic, institutional, regulatory, or credentialing bodies.

The first otolaryngology boot camp, developed at MedStar Georgetown University, focused on preparing junior residents for emergencies. The otolaryngology (ORL) Emergencies Boot Camp curriculum was developed through a needs assessment approach in which common airway, bleeding, and other emergencies were identified.[9] A precourse survey of participating PGY-2 residents found that 87% of novice residents had the greatest anxiety about emergent airway management and establishing a surgical airway.[9] Other concerns included management of hemorrhage, such as epistaxis and postsurgical neck hematoma.

The boot camp purposefully emphasized adult learning principles and was designed to promote hands-on education and directed practice. All 3 domains of learning were included: knowledge, skills, and behaviors.[17] However, every effort was made to accomplish these goals by minimizing lectures and encouraging active participation. Learning objectives for the course and individual stations focus on active learning, critical thinking, and problem solving.

A program based on graduated levels of complexity was developed for learners to progress from simple skills to special skills, and culminating with complex combinations.[7,8,10] Starting the day with simple skills eases the tension, and allows the group to become familiar with the simulation center, staff, and faculty. Furthermore, resident participants are typically from different programs with diverse experiences and varying skill sets. Starting simple with basic airway management, such as bag-valve-mask ventilation, endotracheal intubation, and flexible fiberoptic laryngoscopy can "normalize the playing field" (**Fig. 1**). Focusing a headlight in the oropharynx or nasal cavity to remove a foreign body while coordinating bimanual instrumentation is another valuable skill taught early in the day.

The educational progression follows to more advanced or special skills. Direct laryngoscopy, bronchoscopy, and fiberoptic intubation build on previous airway management techniques. Placement of a surgical airway via cricothyroidotomy and tracheotomy is an essential skill for all otolaryngology first responders. Control of epistaxis with various methods, including anterior and posterior nasal packs, equips residents with the necessary skills to manage even the most difficult nasal hemorrhage cases.

The course concludes with complex scenarios in which residents have the opportunity to combine skills while practicing judgment, communication, and team dynamics. Although facing a real-life emergency scenario is stressful for any otolaryngologist, it can be overwhelming for a junior resident who is encountering such a situation for the first time. Although procedural skills and knowledge are important to navigate an emergency, crisis resource management (CRM) is central to the successful management of all simulation scenarios.[18,19] CRM encompasses the nontechnical skills, such as communication, teamwork, situational awareness, and leadership required to effectively manage all available resources during a health care emergency. The concept originates from Crew Resource Management in the aviation industry. In the 1970s, 70% of airline crashes were found to be due to human error, with failure of teamwork and communication.[4] CRM skills have been increasingly reinforced through medical training, especially in anesthesiology.

Simulation scenarios create an immersive and interactive environment in which learners must think critically, make complex decisions, and manage the clinical situation, often as a team. Throughout the scenarios, the learners use knowledge and procedural skills, but are also required to display teamwork and communication skills while managing hierarchies. At the conclusion of each case, the team debriefs with

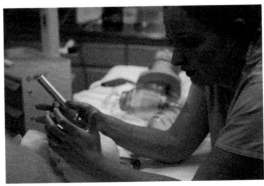

Fig. 1. Faculty demonstrating proper intubation technique on a pediatric mannequin model.

a facilitating faculty member who was involved in the scenario. The discussions allow decompression and solicit reactions from all participants. Details of teamwork, medical management, and lessons learned are explored in a nonthreatening and supportive manner.

At the ORL Emergencies Boot Camp, 2 clinical scenarios are provided, aimed at managing a difficult airway: a case of angioedema requiring a surgical cricothyroidotomy (**Fig. 2**) and a case of a post-thyroidectomy neck hematoma requiring evacuation and airway management. Similar scenarios (post-thyroidectomy neck hematoma and facial fracture requiring definitive surgical airway) are presented at the Western University Boot Camp. These scenarios encourage participants to assemble knowledge and procedural and nontechnical skills to effectively navigate a patient from crisis to definitive and safe management. Many other relevant scenarios could be developed for the same purpose[9,10,13,14] (**Fig. 3**).

The curriculum for the Canadian otolaryngology boot camp at Western University is modeled on the ORL Emergencies Boot Camp and draws residents from across the country. The course targets novice residents in PGY-1 and PGY-2. The emphasis is to transition novice otolaryngology residents from their role as undifferentiated senior medical students to dedicated otolaryngology residents by equipping them with the skill set and confidence to manage commonly encountered as well as rare but life-threatening emergencies. The faculty developed the curriculum for the boot camp at Western University based on common and rare life-threatening emergencies.[13,14] The boot camp emphasizes 2 major emergency categories: (1) complex airway management, including emergent surgical airway control, and (2) managing hemorrhages of the head and neck, such as epistaxis and postoperative neck hematomas.[7–10,14]

RESOURCES

Although boot camps are growing in popularity, many academic programs do not have the infrastructure or institutional support to implement an annual course. Boot camps require significant resources, coordination, and effort. Some of the challenges facing course directors include availability of simulators, simulation space, and experienced faculty.

Simulators

Although otolaryngology-specific simulators are limited, there exists a plethora of task trainers, low-fidelity and high-fidelity mannequins, virtual simulators, and animal and

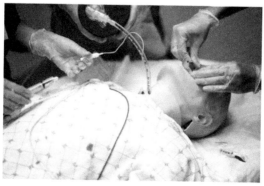

Fig. 2. Angioedema complex scenario managed with placement of surgical airway.

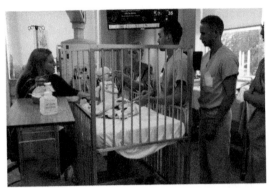

Fig. 3. Residents work through a high-fidelity complex clinical scenario with faculty facilitators to manage a pediatric airway.

other simulator models that can be adapted for our purposes.[20] A recent systematic review identified 64 simulators across the subspecialties of otolaryngology. Luv Javia and Maya Sardesai's article, "Physical Models and Virtual Reality Simulators in Otolaryngology," in this issue, is devoted to physical models and virtual reality simulators in otolaryngology.

Task trainers remain at the very core of clinical skills and procedure instruction and simulation educators rely on them heavily for boot camp education. The goal of a task trainer is to teach the specific steps associated with a particular procedure, and allow repeated practice of the desired skill to become competent. They also allow learners to become familiar with the function and operation of equipment. Task trainers range from low-technology mannequins to low-cost and homemade simulators.

Low-technology airway mannequins have variable fidelity and are designed to teach basic skills, such as mask ventilation. At the ORL Emergencies Boot Camp, skills stations use low-technology mannequins (partial or full body) to practice airway management: bag-valve-mask ventilation, endotracheal intubation, flexible fiberoptic laryngoscopy with intubation, direct laryngoscopy, and bronchoscopy. Infant, child, and adult mannequins are available for all stations (**Fig. 4**). Similarly, low-technology mannequins are used for removal of pharyngeal foreign body and epistaxis management. A fine sewing pin is embedded in the lower pole of the tonsil, and participants must learn coordination of headlight with instruments to identify and remove the

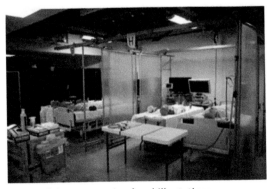

Fig. 4. Infant, child, and adult mannequins for skills stations.

foreign body. The same mannequin is equipped with intravenous (IV) tubing and fake blood to bleed through the nose, allowing residents to practice bimanual dexterity with nasal packing using a nasal speculum, packing material, and a headlight[7,8] (**Fig. 5**).

Low-cost, low-technology simulators can be designed to address a specific skill deficit or need. With some creativity, models can easily be constructed from readily available and reusable materials. A novel and low-cost peritonsillar abscess task trainer uses gelatin and pus-filled water balloons in a cup to teach incision and drainage skills.[21]

High-technology mannequins are programmable and responsive with altering vital signs and palpable pulses. These models are used during the complex scenarios and can be set to exhibit tongue or pharyngeal edema, laryngospasm, or trismus, resulting in a difficult airway. Animal tissues, such as pig feet or cow larynges, are popular in skills training. Local butchers are often willing to give away or sell them at a nominal price. At the ORL Emergencies Boot Camp, pig larynges are used to teach emergency surgical airway procedures. The specimens are stabilized in Styrofoam holders and overlying silicone sheets function as skin. The residents learn laryngotracheal anatomy and perform cricothyroidotomy, tracheotomy, and tracheostomy tube change techniques.[7,8]

The boot camp at Western University innovated several high-fidelity cadaver models as task trainers. By placing IV tubing through the cribriform plate of a formaldehyde-fixed cadaveric head, an epistaxis task trainer was developed. Novice residents can practice focusing their surgical headlamp on a surgical field and coordinating this skill with the use of a nasal speculum and bayonet forceps to pack a nose.[22] Similarly, a cadaver model was developed for learners to practice controlling post-tonsillectomy bleeds or draining a peritonsillar abscess.[23] A glove filled with pudding is placed transcervically within the peritonsillar space of a cadaver head. Multiple learners can practice identifying anatomic landmarks in the pharynx and aspirating. This same cadaver model also was used to practice lateral cantholysis for the treatment of post–sinus surgery orbital hematoma.

Simulation Space/Laboratory

MedStar Georgetown University and Western University are fortunate to have dedicated simulation and surgical laboratory spaces, equipped with a wide range of simulators and supported by experienced simulation staff. In Canada, there are 13 otolaryngology residency programs, and in the United States there are 107.[14] These

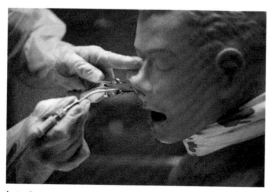

Fig. 5. Epistaxis task trainer.

programs range in size, from 1 to 5 residents per year and may not have the resources to organize and implement such a costly endeavor for a small group of learners.

To get started, programs may consider a smaller-scale effort by using a few clinic, hospital, or operating rooms after hours. The first ORL Emergencies Boot Camp was held on a Saturday in a hospital setting using 3 rooms in a clinic and 3 boardrooms in a conference center. The "dirty" skills station, such as epistaxis control, cricothyroidotomy on pig larynges, and complex scenarios, were conducted in the clinic rooms. The "clean" skills stations, which included basic and airway management on mannequins, were held in the boardrooms. Alternatively, programs within a region may want to share costs and pool resources, such as simulators, staff, and faculty.

Faculty

In addition to the obvious financial and logistical concerns in organizing a boot camp, another practical consideration is the availability of personnel with the appropriate expertise to run the course. Understanding the development of simulation content, creating simulators, and facilitating a debriefing session and validity and reliability concepts are just a few of the relevant aspects currently facing educators. The boot camp planning and implementation can be time and labor intensive, making it difficult for busy faculty to commit to the process. Furthermore, a multitude of staff and faculty is required to operate simulators and ensure appropriate supervision, teaching, and feedback for all the stations and scenarios.

Although most faculty are typically otolaryngologists, the Canadian boot camp incorporates a cross-disciplinary faculty. Anesthesiologists are critical members of the difficult airway team, often working with otolaryngologists in emergent airway situations. Therefore, including anesthesiologists as core faculty in complex airway scenarios teaches collaborative and collegial skills that are invaluable to patient care. Moreover, at Western University, the anesthesiology department regularly trains their residents by using clinical scenario simulations with SimMan (Laederal Medical, Wappingers Fall, NY) and with CRM. Their experience with teaching bag-mask ventilation and laryngoscopy on task trainers, as well as facilitating and debriefing with the simulation scenarios is beneficial.

Regionalization of boot camps ensures an appropriate number of faculty from different institutions with the potential for cross-pollination of various approaches, techniques, and opinions in procedural skills and management of common problems. The ORL Emergencies Boot Camp draws residents and faculty from programs in the mid-Atlantic region, and the Western University Boot Camp hosts residents from all the Canadian otolaryngology programs.[9,14]

OUTCOMES

Simulation-based boot camps are emerging as effective teaching tools. A systematic review of 15 medical education boot camps demonstrated that participants in the boot camp courses had significantly large improvements in clinical skills, knowledge, and confidence.[2] A randomized controlled trial in the United Kingdom concluded that the simulation group had better perception of their learning and scored better on standardized testing for common otolaryngology emergencies when compared with a control group that only had access to didactic lectures.[24]

The course directors of the ORL Emergencies Boot Camp demonstrated improvement of participants' self-perceived knowledge, technical skills, self-confidence, and clinical performance from pre–boot camp to immediately post–boot camp.[9] This improvement was durable at 6 months after the boot camp for all the modules, with the exception of cricothyroidotomy. When these data were further reviewed, Malekzadeh and colleagues[9] found that none of the residents had encountered an urgent airway situation requiring cricothyroidotomy. Without having any further clinical experience with this skill, their self-perceived scores deteriorated.

At the Western University Boot Camp, participants were asked to assess the realism of the models and scenarios. All task trainers were highly rated, and participants were in strong agreement that the models were life-like and of very good quality.[14] The post-tonsillectomy bleed task trainer was found to score less favorably, but still largely considered to be "good" to "very good." Chin and colleagues[13] also assessed participants' self-confidence on a 5-point Likert scale pre–boot camp to immediately post–boot camp. They found the participants' self-confidence to perform tasks increased in all modules, with two-thirds reaching statistical significance. A second survey 1 month after the boot camp revealed that participants attributed their greater confidence in procedural abilities and handling emergency situations to the course. Interestingly, participants did not attribute their improvement in teamwork skills and communication skills with attending the boot camp. Amin and Friedmann[25] designed an advanced airway course specifically for otolaryngology residents. They used objective measures, such as preintervention and postintervention tests and faculty assessment, to assess the effectiveness of their airway simulation modules. After completing the course, the participants' average test score had improved from before the course. Another previously cited randomized study out of the United Kingdom did show that a simulation group had better scores on standardized testing compared with a group that only had the benefit of didactic lectures.[24] However, major limitations of these studies include the absence of control groups and results based on surveys and self-assessments.

Other specialties have used boot camps in training their residents and have demonstrated objective success in resident competency and self-rated confidence. Fann and colleagues[26] reported on their experience with a cardiothoracic training course. They found objective improvement in their cardiothoracic residents' ability to perform vessel anastomosis after the intensive training course. The Society of Neurosurgical Surgeons surveyed their boot camp participants and found that 99% of attendees felt the boot camp had imparted skills and knowledge that improved patient care during their internship.[11,27] Moreover, their follow-up surveys demonstrated that the course material was retained 6 months after the boot camp.[12]

FUTURE DIRECTION

Otolaryngology boot camps across North America and Europe use a wide variety of curricula and a diverse combination of educational tools.[9,14,15] Therefore, resident experiences may differ vastly from program to program. In contrast, our neurosurgery colleagues have elected to standardize boot camps. In Canada, a national neurosurgery boot camp provides training for all PGY-1 residents. Similarly, in the United States, 6 regional neurosurgery boot camps are held during the first month of residency.[11] Residents are assigned precourse reading, and attend standardized lectures and hands-on laboratory sessions at the boot camps. Common clinical scenarios and universal nontechnical skills are emphasized at all the regional boot camps. The course materials are made available online for the residents to access on an ongoing basis during their residency training. The benefits of standardizing an otolaryngology boot camp are numerous. A common curriculum would ensure uniformity of knowledge and skills for all junior residents. Regional simulation centers, equipped with necessary staff and simulation equipment, would be accessible to every residency program. Academic faculty with simulation expertise, dedicated to the education of residents in our specialty, would lead these efforts.

Further studies are needed to examine the impact of introductory boot camps on resident training and patient care. Although participants in both the Western and ORL Emergencies boot camps had improved self-confidence in almost all skills acquired during their respective course, other studies have demonstrated that these benefits were durable up to 1 and 6 months.[14] Other important measures include patients' satisfaction rating of resident physicians, the time required to achieve competency, comparison of skills among trained and untrained residents, and evaluation of patient outcomes.

SUMMARY

Introductory boot camps are being rapidly adopted in otolaryngology and more broadly in medicine. These intensive, 1-day simulation-based courses are designed to allow novice residents the opportunity to practice procedures and manage complex scenarios.

In both objective and subjective measures, boot camps are an effective educational tool. Participants report improved knowledge, technical skills, and self-confidence in managing otolaryngology emergencies. Regionalization of boot camps alleviates the challenges of limited and costly resources. Future studies should focus on the long-term benefits of boot camps, standardization of curricula, and impact on patient outcomes.

REFERENCES

1. Minter RM, Amos KD, Bentz ML, et al. Transition to surgical residency: a multi-institutional study of perceived intern preparedness and the effect of a formal residency preparatory course in the fourth year of medical school. Acad Med 2015; 90(8):1116–24.
2. Blackmore C, Austin J, Lopushinsky SR, et al. Effects of postgraduate medical education "boot camps" on clinical skills, knowledge, and confidence: a meta-analysis. J Grad Med Educ 2014;6(4):643–52.
3. Young JQ, Ranji SR, Wachter RM, et al. "July effect": impact of the academic year-end changes on patient outcomes. Ann Intern Med 2011;155:309.
4. Eidt JF. The aviation model of vascular surgery education. J Vasc Surg 2012; 55(6):1801–9.
5. Fung K. Otolaryngology-head and neck surgery in undergraduate medical education: advances and innovations. Laryngoscope 2015;125(S2):S1–14.
6. Deutsch ES, Wiet GJ, Seidman M, et al. Simulation activity in otolaryngology residencies. Otolaryngol Head Neck Surg 2015;153(2):193–201.
7. Malloy KM, Malekzadeh S, Deutsch ES. Simulation-based otorhinolaryngology emergencies boot camp: part 1: curriculum design and airway skills. Laryngoscope 2014;124(7):1562–5.
8. Malekzadeh S, Deutsch ES, Malloy KM. Simulation-based otorhinolaryngology emergencies boot camp: part 2: special skills using task trainers. Laryngoscope 2014;124(7):1566–9.
9. Malekzadeh S, Malloy KM, Chu EE, et al. ORL emergencies boot camp: using simulation to onboard residents. Laryngoscope 2011;121(10):2114–21.
10. Deutsch ES, Malloy KM, Malekzadeh S. Simulation-based otorhinolaryngology emergencies boot camp: part 3: complex teamwork scenarios and conclusions. Laryngoscope 2014;124(7):1570–2.

11. Selden NR, Origitano TC, Burchiel KJ, et al. A national fundamentals curriculum for neurosurgery PGY1 residents: the 2010 society of neurological surgeons boot camp courses. Neurosurgery 2012;70(4):971–81.
12. Selden NR, Anderson VC, McCartney S, et al. Society of Neurological Surgeons boot camp courses: knowledge retention and relevance of hands-on learning after 6 months of postgraduate year 1 training. J Neurosurg 2013;119(3):796–802.
13. Chin CJ, Chin CA, Roth K, et al. Simulation-based otolaryngology-head and neck surgery boot camp: "how I do it". J Laryngol Otol 2016;130(3):284–90.
14. Chin CJ, Roth K, Rotenberg BW, et al. Emergencies in otolaryngology-head and neck surgery bootcamp: a novel Canadian experience. Laryngoscope 2014; 124(10):2275–80.
15. Smith ME, Trinidade A, Tysome JR. The ENT boot camp: an effective training method for ENT induction. Clin Otolaryngol 2016;41(4):421–4.
16. Hu A, Sardesai MG, Meyer TK. A need for otolaryngology education among primary care providers. Med Educ Online 2012;17(1):1–5.
17. Anderson LW, Krathwohl DR, Airasian PW, et al. A taxonomy of learning teaching and assessing: a revision of bloom's taxonomy of educational objectives. New York: Pearson, Allyn & Bacon; 2001.
18. Boet S, Bould MD, Fung L, et al. Transfer of learning and patient outcome in simulated crisis resource management: a systematic review. Can J Anaesth 2014; 61(6):571–82.
19. Gaba DM, Howard SK, Fish KJ, et al. Simulation-based training in anesthesia crisis resource management (ACRM): a decade of experience. Simul Gaming 2001;32(2):175–93.
20. Javia L, Deutsch ES. A systematic review of simulators in otolaryngology. Otolaryngol Head Neck Surg 2012;147(6):999–1011.
21. Bunting H, Wilson BM, Malloy KM, et al. A novel peritonsillar abscess simulator. Simul Healthc 2015;10:320–5.
22. Scott GM, Roth K, Rotenberg B, et al. Evaluation of a novel high-fidelity epistaxis task trainer. Laryngoscope 2016;126(7):1501–3.
23. Scott GM, Fung K, Roth KE. Novel high-fidelity peritonsillar abscess simulator. Otolaryngol Head Neck Surg 2016;154(4):634–7.
24. Smith ME, Navaratnam A, Jablenska L, et al. A randomized controlled trial of simulation-based training for ear, nose, and throat emergencies. Laryngoscope 2015;125(8):1816–21.
25. Amin MR, Friedmann DR. Simulation-based training in advanced airway skills in an otolaryngology residency program. Laryngoscope 2013;123(3):629–34.
26. Fann JI, Calhoon JH, Carpenter AJ, et al. Simulation in coronary artery anastomosis early in cardiothoracic surgical residency training: the boot camp experience. J Thorac Cardiovasc Surg 2010;139(5):1275–81.
27. Fontes RBV, Selden NR, Byrne RW. Fostering and assessing professionalism and communication skills in neurosurgical education. J Surg Educ 2014;71(6):e83–9.

Using Simulation to Improve Systems

James A. Kearney, MD[a], Ellen S. Deutsch, MD, MS[b,c,d],*

KEYWORDS

- Simulation • Systems • Safety • In situ • Otolaryngology • Quality

KEY POINTS

- Components of the systems that otolaryngologists work within affect their ability to deliver the best care for their patients.
- In situ simulation, particularly when real teams participate in simulations in real patient care areas, can be used to improve the systems that otolaryngologists work within.
- There are many opportunities and techniques that can be used to implement in situ simulation.

As the otolaryngologist on call, you are paged to the emergency department (ED) because of a patient in respiratory distress. You arrive promptly, and find a 56-year-old white male with massive facial edema. He has a history of diabetes and hypertension, and takes insulin and an angiotensin-converting enzyme inhibitor. He has no known drug allergies. The ED physicians have administered epinephrine with no significant improvement. Two attempts at intubation have been unsuccessful. You recognize that he has medication-related angioedema. The patient is struggling to breathe and his oxygen saturation is 92%.

Planning to perform cricothyrotomy, you request a scalpel. The nurse hands you an unusual scalpel; it is a safety scalpel (**Fig. 1**). You palpate the patient's neck to find surgical landmarks, and prepare to make an incision, but the blade is covered by a safety sheath and you fumble to try to retract the sheath. The patient's oxygen saturation is now 87%. You eventually get the blade exposed, nearly cutting yourself in the process, and make your incision. You enter the airway - success! You ask for a Yankauer suction and one arrives in your hand, but it does not seem to work, although you can

Conflicts of interest: None.

[a] Pennsylvania Hospital, University of Pennsylvania Health System, Perelman School of Medicine at the University of Pennsylvania, 800 Walnut Street, 18th Floor, Philadelphia, PA 19107, USA; [b] Department of Anesthesiology and Critical Care Medicine, Children's Hospital of Philadelphia, Perelman School of Medicine at the University of Pennsylvania, Philadelphia, PA, USA; [c] Pennsylvania Patient Safety Authority, Harrisburg, PA, USA; [d] ECRI Institute, 5200 Butler Pike, Plymouth Meeting, PA 19462, USA

* Corresponding author. ECRI Institute, 5200 Butler Pike, Plymouth Meeting, PA 19462.

E-mail address: edeutsch@ecri.org

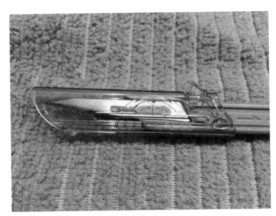

Fig. 1. Close-up of safety sheath on disposable scalpel.

hear the sound of the suction. What is the problem? Troubleshooting reveals that the suction canister is cracked. The respiratory therapist grabs the suction canister from the next bay and replaces the cracked one. Although this is accomplished fairly quickly, it has been a distraction, and you can hear the pitch of the pulse oximeter getting lower, as the patient's oxygen saturation continues to decrease. Nevertheless, you insert a tracheotomy tube and, with practiced fluency, you pull out the obturator, insert the inner cannula, and attach a CO_2 detector, which confirms correct placement of the tracheostomy tube. The respiratory therapist promptly connects supplemental oxygen, the patient appears to be more comfortable, and his oxygen saturation improves.

Because this issue is focused on simulation, it may not be surprising to learn that the same patient may appear in the ED again and again, and is a high-technology manikin. Many of the articles in this issue address ways in which simulation can be used to enhance the capabilities of individuals and of teams. However, the story that unfolds during this simulation provides examples of how the environment in which health care is delivered also affects clinicians' ability to provide safe, effective, and timely care.

This angioedema simulation may have been designed to enhance the teamwork skills of the participants, and identifying the equipment problems was serendipitous, or this simulation may have been an intentional system probe, conducted in situ (eg, in a real ED) to identify problems before real patients might be affected. In either event, in addition to providing an opportunity for the participants to reflect on the medical management of the simulated patient, the debriefing after the simulation provides an opportunity to acknowledge and begin to mitigate the equipment problems.

HOW DO SYSTEM COMPONENTS AFFECT CLINICIANS' ABILITY TO CARE FOR THEIR PATIENTS?

Attempts to understand and improve health care delivery often focus on the characteristics of the patient and the characteristics of the health care providers, but larger systems surround and integrate with patients and providers; components of these systems can support or interfere with efforts to provide optimal health care. Health care delivery is a sociotechnical system in which multiple agents and system components affect, and are affected by, other agents and other system components.[1,2] In the case of the patient with angioedema described in the beginning of this article, the otolaryngologist had the knowledge and skills to control the patient's airway, but had to use an unfamiliar scalpel.

The attempt to suction the patient's airway was an appropriate action, but the necessary equipment was broken and this interfered with the team's ability to provide the best care possible for the patient. The problems with the scalpel and the suction canister were threats to the ability to provide safe care for the patient. Presuming that the equipment problems had not been recognized before the equipment was needed, and had not previously contributed to harm for a patient, they were latent safety threats (LST). In medicine, LSTs have been defined as system-based threats to patient safety that can materialize at any time[3] and are previously unrecognized by health care providers, unit directors, or hospital administration.[4]

At first, fixing this problem of receiving a scalpel that is difficult to use seems to be simple, because these scalpels could be removed from stock and replaced by scalpels that are easier to use. However, the decision about which scalpel to stock can be used to show how the relationship between system components is extraordinarily complex, adaptive, fluid, and dynamic.[1,2] Maybe the difficult scalpel was selected for use by the health care facility because it was less expensive, because the organization had entered into a purchasing contract to help manage external financial pressures. Maybe the difficult scalpel was selected because it was thought to be safer for health care workers, with less chance of worker injury. Maybe the difficult scalpel was selected because providers in another department found it preferable, and the facility saw value in standardizing supplies across the organization, which could make purchasing, storage, and restocking easier. Perhaps there are other factors that were integrated into the purchasing or stocking decision.

The broad and diverse range of system components that interact and affect health care delivery have been articulated by several investigators, including Carayon and colleagues,[5] Vincent and Amalberti,[6] Harrison and colleagues,[7] and Sittig and Singh.[8] Components of health care delivery that interact in complex ways include the work environment and workflow, patient outcomes, processes and protocols, institutional context and financial pressures, organizational management, task factors, and technology and technology infrastructure and interfaces.

The Institute of Medicine (IOM) report *To Err is Human* stated that "medical errors are not a result of isolated individual actions but rather faulty systems, processes, and conditions that lead people to make mistakes."[9] In light of the complexity of health care delivery, understanding and improving the systems, processes, and conditions that are involved in health care is also complex, and many approaches have been developed. Often improvement processes attempt to understand patient care in response to undesired outcomes, such as by conducting root cause analyses and departmental morbidity and mortality conferences. The emerging capabilities of so-called, "big data" aggregated from numerous individual episodes of health care delivery, may reveal patterns that are not always evident from individual patient experiences. Information may be gathered from focus groups and meetings of stakeholders, from chart review using processes such as trigger tools,[10,11] and from analysis of aggregate data; these processes can be considered, respectively, as work-as-imagined,[12] work-as-documented, and work-as-abstracted. Each of these sources of analysis helps provide information about some components of health care delivery, and each is unavoidably incomplete. Similarly, Six Sigma, LEAN and other techniques may be used in efforts to enhance health care delivery value. Work-as-simulated provides a valuable complementary perspective, functioning as both a technique for process improvement and a method of education. The IOM, the Joint Commission, and the Agency for Healthcare Research and Quality recommend medical simulation as an important safe practice intervention to reduce errors and risks associated with the process of care.[13–15]

WHAT IS IN SITU SIMULATION AND WHY IS IT IMPORTANT?

The Merriam-Webster Dictionary defines in situ as meaning "in the natural or original position or place."[16] Work-as-simulated, using simulation in situ, focuses on team responses and systems performance rather than individual knowledge, performance, or technical skills. Real teams participating in simulations in real care settings can help bridge the gap between work-as-imagined (work as it is presumed or thought to occur),[12] and work as it really occurs. The larger the number or type of in situ conditions included in the simulation, the greater the fidelity of the simulation compared with real work. For example, when simulating a trauma resuscitation in a patient with rapid hemorrhage, it may be worthwhile to involve blood bank personnel. LSTs that could affect activation of the massive transfusion protocol may be identified at any point of the activation process, and could potentially be mitigated before patient harm occurs. In aviation, and other high-hazard fields, the inclusion of the entire crew, including ground and maintenance personnel, was beneficial in attempts to optimize communication and teamwork skills.[17] Patterson and colleagues[18] describe in situ simulations as "Simulations that occur in the actual clinical environment and whose participants are on-duty clinical providers during their actual workday." The more closely work as simulated in situ approaches work as it is really done, the more valuable the information that can be derived, and the more likely that iterative improvement processes can identify and mitigate unintended consequences of process changes.

In situ simulation complements simulation conducted in simulation centers. The target audience and objectives overlap but each training environment has advantages and disadvantages. Training based at a simulation center is often best suited for skill acquisition for novices and less experienced learners. Beginners benefit from the dedicated simulation center environment, in which there is less pressure and a greater opportunity to make mistakes outside of a clinical area. In situ simulation allows intermediate and experienced practitioners to review and reinforce their skills and to problem-solve in the clinical environment.[18,19] Simulation centers may also offer advantages for some types of research that require standardized conditions.[20]

Even in simulations designed solely as intentional system probes, participant learning is inevitable. Kolb and colleagues'[21] theory of experiential learning provides a rationale for conducting in situ simulation from the perspective of both the educator and the participant. The theory posits that effective adult learning relies on concrete experiences, reflection on these experiences, and active experimentation so that new ideas and concepts can be used in practice.[21] In situ training creates an activated learner by putting the adult learner in an authentic environment[22] and demonstrating the clinical relevance of the new skill.[17]

In situ simulation helps to fill the gap between knowledge and practice. Clinical care continues to lag behind clinical research, with some estimates indicating that it takes 17 years for 14% of research discoveries to be translated into practice.[23] Studies repeatedly show that front-line clinical care deviates from compliance with evidence-based policies and guidance.[24,25] In situ simulation can serve as a medium to understand the degree to which management is evidence based, and debriefing can be useful to identify reasons for irregularities in care, including discordance with evidence, and to suggest potential solutions.[17]

CURRENT STATE OF IN SITU SIMULATION IN OTOLARYNGOLOGY

In situ simulation is not broadly used by otolaryngologists at present. In 2011, 43 of 104 otolaryngology residency training programs responded to a survey about simulation; only 28.6% of respondents said that in situ simulation resources were available at their institution, although 50% of the respondents were using simulation for systems improvement.[26] Review for this article showed sparse literature devoted to in situ simulation specific to otolaryngology, but several publications present applications of in situ simulation that could be relevant for many otolaryngology programs.

Johnson and colleagues[27] describe concerns generated by delays in the management of a child who presented to their ED with critical airway obstruction caused by foreign body aspiration. Although the patient's eventual outcome was good, the event prompted a review and revision of the institution's system of care for any child with critical airway obstruction who might present to the ED. Otolaryngologists and simulationists collaborated to create a simulation of a 4-year-old child with foreign body aspiration. The simulations took place in situ, in the ED, where participants interacted with a high-technology manikin and viewed a video of a real child in respiratory distress with audible stridor and visible retractions. The first set of 6 simulations was used to assess the existing system of care. Based on information derived from the simulations, several process changes were implemented, such as developing a critical airway response team and developing an airway cart with specialized equipment. A final set of 6 simulations was conducted, showing improved timeliness and quality of care for simulated patients. In addition to the education provided to team members, the in situ simulations revealed 13 unique LSTs, such as the lack of a needle cricothyroidotomy kit in the ED, which were then addressed.[27] This experience shows how in situ simulation can reveal information, such as response times or misplaced equipment, that is less likely to be identified using other investigatory processes.

In preparation for opening a new satellite ED, Geis and colleagues[28] conducted a variety of in situ simulations, including simulation of a posttonsillectomy hemorrhage, to allow members of newly formed teams to practice working together, and to identify LSTs. Most of the LSTs identified before the site was opened for actual patient care involved equipment or resources; the remainder involved medications and personnel. Findings included impaired access to airway equipment and lack of surgical airway management equipment, as well as insufficient oxygen flow to support bag-mask ventilation of 2 patients simultaneously and lack of specific resuscitation equipment. Of the 37 identified LSTs, 32 (86%) were resolved or managed before opening the facility.[28]

Volk and colleagues[29] implemented an interprofessional in situ simulation course, addressing the management of a patient in an operating room (OR) with an evolving medical problem. Compared with their previous courses conducted in a simulation center, the interprofessional in situ course was more realistic, supported improved team dynamics, and had logistical advantages for the residents. Although the intended purpose of the course was to teach decision-making, teamwork, and crisis resource management skills, LSTs were identified during the in situ simulations. The switches that activate emergency responses were difficult to locate because of poor signage and more than the usual amount of equipment in the OR; this finding prompted the OR administration to improve the signage.[22,29]

Literature describing in situ simulation in otolaryngology[22,27,29] has come primarily from institutions with a commitment to in situ simulation across multiple disciplines. Because of the team nature of in situ training it would be challenging for otolaryngology alone to drive the process of designing and implementing multidisciplinary or interprofessional scenarios relevant for otolaryngologists. An ideal approach would be for an institution to commit to this process across disciplines and then have an otolaryngology champion to help develop and run otolaryngology-focused simulations.

ADVANTAGES OF IN SITU SIMULATION

The examples of system improvements generated by in situ otolaryngology simulations are in line with experiences in other specialties. In situ simulation allows identification of LSTs before patients are harmed. Patterson and colleagues[4] identified 73 LSTs during 90 in situ ED simulations conducted over 1 year, averaging 1 LST for every 1.2 simulations performed. This rate was dramatically higher than their previous rate of identifying an average of 1 LST for every 7 simulations performed in their simulation center.

Recreating patient care events, including sentinel events, to allow for root cause or other analysis in the clinical environment in which the event occurred may reveal information that would not have been evident using only interviews and focus group processes.

Conducting simulations in situ can support program development without the expense of building a simulation center, thus lowering a barrier to implementing simulation. In situ opportunities can be more cost-efficient for staff learners because they do not need to devote separate time to go to a simulation center and require replacement staffing while they train off their units.[22]

In situ simulation has the potential to allow for simulation as a tool for quality improvement (QI) and patient safety in institutions outside of academic centers. In situ simulation can also be portable; mobile simulation has potential to allow community and rural health care sites to use simulation.[30]

In situ simulation may make it easier to gather and train intact, interprofessional teams if the sessions occur while they are already on duty together. Training is more effective when health care teams rehearse communication and nontechnical skills in their normal clinical setting, using real medical equipment, and learners function in their actual professional roles.[31]

HIGH-STAKES LOW-FREQUENCY EVENTS PERTINENT TO OTOLARYNGOLOGY

Patient conditions that are infrequent but may have serious consequences provide useful material for in situ simulations. Examples of system findings that have been identified during in situ simulations include an inability to obtain blood for transfusion in a case of massive hemorrhage because the protocol to obtain blood required paperwork that was not available at the point of care; general lack of knowledge about where to obtain ice and how to dilute sodium dantrolene during a simulation of malignant hyperthermia; and lack of intubation medications for a patient whose condition deteriorated in the postoperative care unit (**Fig. 2**). Examples of medical conditions that could be simulated to generate insight into system capabilities are listed in **Box 1**.

LOGISTICS OF IN SITU SIMULATION

First, set goals and objectives. One key to a successful in situ simulation is to determine specific learning objectives during the planning stage and align these objectives with organizational QI and patient safety goals. Analysis and documentation of in situ simulation findings can be structured to make their relevance to organizational goals explicit. Learning objectives should be observable, measurable, and meaningful.[30] Broad categories of objectives include:

- Instruction to develop and facilitate application of cognitive, technical, or teamwork competencies
- Assessment of performance or a health care delivery process
- Diagnosis of potential risks or system defects[19]

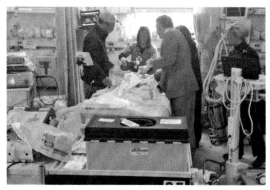

Fig. 2. In situ simulation of a patient with an expanding neck hematoma and airway compromise following anterior cervical discectomy and spinal fusion, in the postanesthesia care unit.

Another key to success is providing feedback to participants about plans to address LSTs that are identified and progress toward resolving them. In situ simulation can make LSTs explicitly visible, whether the LSTs were intentionally sought or discovered serendipitously. If feedback is not provided about resolving identified issues it can lead to frustration and anger that the organization is committed only to patient safety on the

---

Box 1
High-stakes low-frequency medical conditions that could provide stem stories for informative simulations

Inability to intubate or ventilate, requiring an emergency surgical airway

Oropharyngeal hemorrhage with loss of airway

Obstructing endobronchial foreign body or clot

Carotid blowout with massive blood loss

Tension pneumothorax

Anaphylaxis

Airway fire in the OR

Power outage in the OR

Anaphylaxis in the OR or in the office

Malignant hyperthermia

Massive epistaxis with loss of the airway

Laryngospasm with negative pressure pulmonary edema in PACU or the OR

Massive pulmonary embolus in the OR

Air embolus in the OR

Carotid injury during sphenoid surgery

Occluded or dislodged tracheotomy tube

Rapidly expanding neck hematoma

Abbreviation: PACU, postanesthesia care unit.

backs of hypervigilant individuals, rather than to robust supporting systems.[18] For example, in the case presented at the beginning of this article, feedback to participants that broken suction canisters are being methodically identified and replaced would contribute to reassuring participants that safety is taken seriously by the organization.

WHO

An in situ simulation is typically led by an experienced simulationist and usually requires at least 2 or 3 people to set up, run the simulation, and then debrief. Typical requirements include a simulationist who can facilitate designing, implementing, and debriefing the simulation; a simulator operator if a high-technology manikin is used; a content expert; and a local champion. Many times 1 person can fulfill more than 1 of these roles, but it is rare to need fewer than 2 people. Depending on the objectives of the simulation, involvement from ancillary services such as pharmacy, blood bank, and information technology (IT) may be appropriate. Involvement of unit supervisors is critical in setting goals and objectives, judging whether the scheduled time for the simulation will not interfere with real patient care, and in assessing the effectiveness of the simulation.[18] Involving staff from QI/patient safety is valuable to document the LSTs uncovered and to make plans to correct them. Personnel with additional skills, such as human factors experts, anthropologists, or informaticists, may provide additional perspectives and insights.

WHAT

The degree to which real medications, blood products, equipment, supplies, technology, or other resources are integrated into the simulation affects the fidelity, or realism, of the simulation. Thoughtful decisions must be made about which components of actual patient care processes should be incorporated. For example, learning endoscopy with an out-of-date, discarded endoscopy tower does not provide the same understanding of the equipment and quality of learning as using a contemporary model, and does not provide the opportunity to identify LSTs that may be related to specific equipment or equipment setups. In contrast, when using real medications and blood products, the cost of wasted medication and the potential to waste human blood products must be considered. The use of simulated medications (eg, expired or fake medications) may save money but introduces a potential to mix these medications with real medications and could create a patient safety issue.

In situ simulation may involve the use of real equipment. The in situ simulation leaders need to protect equipment from damage, and ensure that participation does not preclude a response to real patient emergencies that could arise during a simulation.

The cooperation of the IT department can facilitate the creation of an electronic medical record for a simulated patient; this is an increasingly important component of simulations because electronic interfaces have become ubiquitous in patient care processes.

At the conclusion of the simulation, simulation personnel should ensure that supplies and equipment that were used are sufficiently restocked and replaced.

WHERE

In situ simulations can be held almost anywhere within or around a health care facility. Typical locations include:

- ORs
- EDs, including trauma and resuscitation bays

- Intensive care units
- Labor and delivery suites
- Medical or surgical inpatient care units
- Outpatient clinics or offices

Children's Hospital of Philadelphia has added simulation infrastructure to a real OR by adding a control room containing computers for high-technology manikins, video recording and communication equipment, and a window into the OR.[32] Booms within the OR were modified to provide cables and other resources for manikins. Use of the room typically occurs during early morning educational time, which is shared by surgery, anesthesia, and nursing, or on weekends.

With portable simulators, simulations can also be held in sites where patient care may be needed during uncommon situations, such as in stuck elevators, parking lots or garages, or ambulances, as well as sites where employees may have medical emergencies, such as administrative areas and supply rooms.

WHEN

It is easiest for the simulation team to run in situ simulations during day shift on weekdays, but health care is a 24/7/365 process. Research has shown that patient outcomes are worse for patients admitted on weekends.[33,34] Perhaps off-hour simulation will have the highest yield in patient safety improvement. Strategies to assist in training off-hour personnel include running simulations just before or after shift changes.[30] Patient census is often lower in the early morning, and simulations scheduled for this time of day (eg, before 7 AM) might facilitate participation by night shift personnel; simulations scheduled for early Mondays might also allow participation of weekend personnel.

There are pros and cons to conducting in situ simulations as announced or unannounced. Scheduled in situ simulations allow for a prebrief to prepare individuals unfamiliar with simulation with an introduction to the concept and the parameters, to set expectations and allay anxiety. An announced in situ simulation also allows participants to prepare by addressing knowledge or skill gaps and familiarizing themselves with equipment or processes.

Unscheduled in situ simulation has the advantage of real-time assessment of environment and processes, but runs the risk of generating resentment from disrupting the normal work day and creating a poor attitude toward simulation. It may be best to familiarize participants by introducing in situ simulations to a unit or institution on a scheduled basis.[30]

HOW

The following list includes suggestions for factors to consider when organizing an in situ simulation:

1. Identify goals and objectives; be specific, define what will be measured.
2. Identify location and scenario content.
3. Meet with involved parties to plan, including managers, pharmacy, IT, blood bank, QI, patient safety officers, and others as appropriate.
4. Designate location for debriefing and ensure enough time to debrief.
5. Choose date and make arrangements for simulation personnel and equipment.
6. Ensure that simulation will not put real patients at risk by consulting with the unit manager just before the simulation. Be prepared to cancel if the manager deems patient volume or acuity to be too high to allow the simulation.

7. On day of event warn patients and visitors that a simulation is occurring. Patients and families are generally very supportive and appreciate the value of the training, but sensitive preparation is helpful.[18]
8. Run the simulation and debrief in a limited and predictable time framework to minimize the disruption to workflow. Initially simulations may take longer because of their novelty, and the need to set the desired tone and parameters, but, with increased experience, the duration of the simulations, including the debriefings, may become shorter.
9. Ask QI/patient safety to give feedback to the involved parties about issues identified and mitigation plans. Request that formal feedback be given to involved parties at a defined follow-up interval (eg, 3–6 months) to let participants know that their involvement in the simulation made a difference.

CHALLENGES TO IN SITU SIMULATION

In situ simulations are time intensive for clinicians to plan and run. They are also more time intensive for simulation technicians because equipment transport, setup, and breakdown often take longer than similar tasks in a simulation center. Mobile setup units can decrease setup time.[30] Obtaining buy-in from leadership is invaluable.

In situ simulations are subject to abrupt cancellation if a unit has high patient acuity or census. Last-minute cancellations can result in wasted time for several individuals involved in planning the simulation, and investigators have quoted a 10% to 30% cancellation rate.[4,27,31] However, a willingness to cancel a simulation because of patient care needs is necessary for success.[18]

Patterson and colleagues[4] implemented an in situ simulation project in an ED to promote the identification of LSTs, and the cancellation rate decreased over time as the simulations matured. Approximately half way through their project, the ED leadership thought that the training was sufficiently valuable to require mandatory participation by all ED care providers.

Clinical staff have limited time for simulation; bringing the simulations to the staff decreases the need for transit time, and may allow simulations to be incorporated into clinical schedules in creative ways. Simulations can be constrained to an hour, a half an hour, or even less. Patterson and colleagues[18] describe a 17-minute framework, including a 10-minute simulation immediately followed by a 7-minute debriefing.

Postsimulation surveys, often used for continuous QI of the simulations, can be used to assess the perceived value of performing the simulations during the workday, any negative impact on actual patient care, and any additional issues that participants might not have been comfortable voicing during the debriefing.[4] Surveys can be completed at the time of the event, or sent to participants later; the timing may affect completion rates.

Performance anxiety of health care providers can be a major hurdle. A goal of simulation is to provide a safe learning environment but confidentiality may be difficult to preserve in the hospital setting. During team training, an individual's clinical weaknesses and knowledge gaps may be revealed to teammates who later need to trust each other and work together.[30] Therefore, it should be made clear to participants that the intent of the simulation is to probe for LSTs, so attention can be focused away from the performance of individuals and toward understanding and improving the health care delivery process and environment.

Additional challenges can be diverse and are not always entirely predictable. Locations for computers and compressors needed for some high-technology manikins may be limited. Wireless connections that functioned perfectly well during practice sessions or equipment testing may fail to function during the simulation. Rehearsal of the scenario may not be possible until just before the simulation, if at all. During the simulation, participants may be distracted by pagers, phone calls, and patient care responsibilities,[30] but these reflect the realities of actual patient care. Debriefing space may be limited and not sufficiently private[30]; debriefing near or even in the space where simulations were conducted is usually preferable to traveling some distance within the facility to debrief because much of the learning from the simulation may be diffused as participants chat en route to the debriefing site.

Debriefing

A respectful, supportive, and skilled debriefing is essential to establish a constructive tone and process, to model desirable behaviors, and to optimize learning from each simulation. Although the content of an in situ simulation may differ from a simulation focused primarily on teamwork skills and knowledge, the principles of debriefing in situ simulations are essentially the same and are addressed in Sarah N. Bowe and colleagues' article, "Facilitation and Debriefing in Simulation Education," in this issue. Debriefing is mentioned in this article only to reemphasize its critical importance.

Systems Issues Identified

Systems issues relevant to otolaryngology that have been identified either during otolaryngology simulations or by other investigators[17,18,30,31] are listed in **Table 1**.

PEARLS FOR SUCCESS

- Start with scheduled in situ simulations to introduce the concept.
- Given the time pressures associated with in situ simulation, the debriefing in this setting is by necessity brief and concise.[18]
- The key to success is less related to the site or technology, and more to the faculty that deliver it.[35]

SUMMARY

Health care is delivered in a uniquely complex sociotechnical system[20] and surgeons work in one of the most complex sociotechnical systems in existence. Optimizing the health care knowledge and skills of individuals and teams is essential, but not sufficient. The IOM recommendations to prevent errors include "designing systems that make it hard for people to do the wrong thing and easy for people to do the right thing"[9]; this system approach can be expanded to enhance many aspects of patient safety. "Poor designs set the workforce up to fail, regardless of how hard they try. If we want safer, higher-quality care, we will need to have redesigned systems of care."[36]

In situ simulation is a versatile tool that can be used to expose and help to mitigate LSTs. Simulation can be used throughout the development or modification of health care processes, starting with architectural planning and continuing through ongoing, continuous QI. LSTs may be difficult for the people working in a system to notice because the errors may be "hidden in the design of routine processes,"[9] and in situ simulation may bring these LSTs to light. Even the need to cancel a planned simulation because of limited human or equipment resources provides information and can be understood as an indication that the system involved may not have sufficient margin, and patient care may be at risk, if any additional system stressor develops. In situ simulations provide a mechanism to refocus attention on the environment, protocols, technologies, equipment, and other factors that interact with and affect health care

Table 1
Systems issues with relevance for otolaryngology that have been identified during in situ simulations

Communication	• Reluctance to think out loud • Lack of closed loop communication • Lack of communication caused by assumption of knowledge
Medication issues	• Lack of speedy access • Lack of knowledge deficits about contraindications, dose, route of administration
Environment	• Stock not available
Devices/ equipment	• Staff unaware of location of equipment • Staff unfamiliar with equipment • Batteries removed or dead • Electronic medical record issues • Elevators too slow to get personnel, equipment, or patient to needed location
Staffing/roles	• Staff unavailable • Lack of clarity of staff roles in crisis situation
Protocols	• Insufficient knowledge of protocols • Lack of difficult airway alert • Communication barriers delay summoning emergency support

delivery. Simulation, particularly in situ simulation, is a powerful technique that can be used to help understand and improve health care delivery; to expose LSTs; and to model respectful, constructive approaches to developing, testing, and improving health care delivery processes.

REFERENCES

1. Dekker S. Drift into failure from hunting broken components to understanding complex systems. Farnham (United Kingdom): Ashgate; 2011.
2. Vincent C. Patient safety. 2nd edition. West Sussex (United Kingdom): John Wiley; 2010.
3. Alfredsdottir H, Bjornsdottir K. Nursing and patient safety in the operating room. J Adv Nurs 2008;61(1):29–37.
4. Patterson MD, Geis GL, Falcone RA, et al. In situ simulation: detection of safety threats and teamwork training in a high risk emergency department. BMJ Qual Saf 2013;22(6):468–77.
5. Carayon P, Schoofs Hundt A, Karsh BT, et al. Work system design for patient safety: the SEIPS model. Qual Saf Health Care 2006;15(Suppl 1):i50–8.
6. Vincent C, Amalberti R. Safer healthcare strategies for the real world. Cham (Switzerland): SpringerOpen; 2016.
7. Harrison MI, Henriksen K, Hughes RG. Improving the health care work environment: a sociotechnical systems approach. Jt Comm J Qual Patient Saf 2007; 33(11 Suppl):3–6.
8. Sittig DF, Singh H. A new sociotechnical model for studying health information technology in complex adaptive healthcare systems. Qual Saf Health Care 2010;19(Suppl 3):68–74.
9. Institute of Medicine Committee on Quality of Health Care in America. To err is human: building a safer health system. Washington, DC: National Academy Press; 1999.

10. Mattsson TO, Knudsen JL, Lauritsen J, et al. Assessment of the global trigger tool to measure, monitor and evaluate patient safety in cancer patients: reliability concerns are raised. BMJ Qual Saf 2013;22(7):571–9.

11. Stockwell DC, Bisarya H, Classen DC, et al. A trigger tool to detect harm in pediatric inpatient settings. Pediatrics 2015;135(6):1036–42.

12. Hollnagel E, Wears R, Braithwaite J. From safety-I to safety-II: a white paper. 2015.

13. Shojania KG, Duncan BW, McDonald KM, et al. Making health care safer: a critical analysis of patient safety practices. Evidence Report: Technology Assessment (Summary). Agency for Healthcare Research and Quality (AHRQ); 2001.

14. IOM (Institute of Medicine). Measuring the impact of interprofessional education on collaborative practice and patient outcomes. 2015.

15. Joint commission online. 2014. Available at: http://www.jointcommission.org/assets/1/23/jconline_October_22_14.pdf. Accessed December 11, 2016.

16. In situ. Available at: https://www.merriam-webster.com/dictionary/in%20situ. Accessed December 3, 2016.

17. Guise J, Mladenovic J. In situ simulation: identification of systems issues. Semin Perinatol 2013;37(3):161–5.

18. Patterson MD, Blike GT, Nadkarni VM. In situ simulation: challenges and results. In: Henriksen K, Battles JB, Keyes MA, et al, editors. Advances in patient safety: new directions and alternative approaches (vol. 3: performance and tools) publication no 08-0034-3. Rockville (MD): Agency for Healthcare Research and Quality; 2008. Available at: http://wwwahrq.gov/downloads/pub/advances2/vol3/advances-patterson_48.pdf. Accessed November 8, 2016.

19. Groom JA. Creating new solutions to the simulation puzzle. Simul Healthc 2009; 4(3):131–4.

20. Deutsch ES, Dong Y, Halamek LP, et al. Leveraging health care simulation technology for human factors research: closing the gap between lab and bedside. Hum Factors 2016;58(7):1082–95.

21. Kolb AY, Kolb DA, editors. The Kolb learning style inventory - version 3.1 2005 technical specifications. Philadelphia: HayGroup Experience Based Learning Systems; 2005.

22. Weinstock PH, Kappus LJ, Garden A, et al. Simulation at the point of care: reduced-cost, in situ training via a mobile cart. Pediatr Crit Care Med 2009; 10(2):176–81.

23. Balas E, Boren S. Managing clinical knowledge for health care improvement. In: van Bemmel JH, McCray AT, editors. Yearbook of medical informatics. Stuttgart (Germany): Schattauer Verlagsgesellschaft mbH; 2000. p. 65–70.

24. Cabana MD, Rand CS, Powe NR, et al. Why don't physicians follow clinical practice guidelines? A framework for improvement. JAMA 1999;282(15):1458–65.

25. Lomas J, Anderson GM, Domnick-Pierre K, et al. Do practice guidelines guide practice? the effect of a consensus statement on the practice of physicians. N Engl J Med 1989;321(19):1306–11.

26. Deutsch ES, Wiet GJ, Seidman M, et al. Simulation activity in otolaryngology residencies. Otolaryngol Head Neck Surg 2015;153(2):193–201.

27. Johnson K, Geis G, Oehler J, et al. Simulation to implement a novel system of care for pediatric critical airway obstruction. Arch Otolaryngol Head Neck Surg 2012;138(10):907–11.

28. Geis GL, Pio B, Pendergrass TL, et al. Simulation to assess the safety of new healthcare teams and new facilities. Simul Healthc 2011;6(3):125–33.

29. Volk MS, Ward J, Irias N, et al. Using medical simulation to teach crisis resource management and decision-making skills to otolaryngology housestaff. Otolaryngol Head Neck Surg 2011;145(1):35–42.

30. Maa T, Heimberg E, Reid JR. In situ simulation. In: Grant VJ, Cheng A, editors. Comprehensive healthcare simulation: pediatrics. Switzerland: Springer International; 2016. p. 153–63.

31. Wheeler DS, Geis G, Mack EH, et al. High-reliability emergency response teams in the hospital: improving quality and safety using in situ simulation training. BMJ Qual Saf 2013;22(6):507–14.

32. Lockman JL, Ambardekar AP, Deutsch ES. Optimizing education with in situ simulation. In: Palaganas JC, Maxworthy JC, Epps CA, et al, editors. Defining excellence in simulation programs. Philadelphia: Wolters Kluwer; 2015. p. 90–8.

33. Kostis WJ, Demissie K, Marcella SW, et al. Weekend versus weekday admission and mortality from myocardial infarction. N Engl J Med 2007;356(11):1099–109.

34. Shaheen AAM, Kaplan GG, Myers RP. Weekend versus weekday admission and mortality from gastrointestinal hemorrhage caused by peptic ulcer disease. Clin Gastroenterol Hepatol 2009;7(3):303–10.

35. Weinstock P. Weathering the perfect storm: a deeper look at simulation applied to pediatric critical care. Pediatr Crit Care Med 2012;13(2):226–7.

36. Institute of Medicine, editor. Crossing the quality chasm: a new health system for the 21st century. Washington, DC: National Academy of Sciences; 2000.

The Economics of Surgical Simulation

Noel Jabbour, MD, MS[a],*, Carl H. Snyderman, MD, MBA[b,c]

KEYWORDS

- Surgical simulation • Economics • Surgical education • Residency training costs
- Cost analysis

KEY POINTS

- There are massive hidden costs in the current paradigm of surgical training related to increased operative times for procedures with resident involvement and costs of medical errors.
- Shifting training outside of the operating room through simulation can potentially improve patient safety, minimize learning time to achieve competency, and increase operative efficiency.
- Investment in surgical simulation has the potential to reduce costs to health care systems through improved operating room efficiency and reduction of medical errors.

INTRODUCTION

The traditional method of training surgeons has been threatened by 3 coincident challenges—an increased interest in patient safety in the operating room (OR), a compressed surgical training experience owing to duty-hour regulations, and increasing costs of operative care with decreased reimbursement. As surgical educators, each of these "problems" can be viewed as potential opportunities to improve the method by which we train future surgeons by shifting the learning outside of the OR environment into more effective learning environments that improve patient safety, minimize learning time required to obtain competency, and increase operative efficiency. This article explores each of these "problems" and the potential opportunity that each provides for simulation training from an economic perspective. What are the hidden costs

Disclosure Statement: The authors have nothing to disclose.
[a] Division of Pediatric Otolaryngology, Children's Hospital of Pittsburgh of UPMC, University of Pittsburgh School of Medicine, 4401 Penn Avenue, Faculty Pavilion, 7th Floor, Pittsburgh, PA 15224, USA; [b] Department of Otolaryngology, Center for Cranial Base Surgery, The Eye & Ear Institute, University of Pittsburgh School of Medicine, 200 Lothrop Street, Suite 500, Pittsburgh, PA 15213, USA; [c] Department of Neurological Surgery, Center for Cranial Base Surgery, The Eye & Ear Institute, University of Pittsburgh School of Medicine, 200 Lothrop Street, Suite 500, Pittsburgh, PA 15213, USA
* Corresponding author.
E-mail address: JabbourN@chp.edu

of surgical training? How do we pay for surgical simulation? What will it cost… or will it actually save our system money?

CURRENT CONTEXT AND RESPONSIBILITY AS SURGICAL EDUCATORS

As surgical educators, we have a duty to teach to competence. This duty is not only to our trainees, but also to society. Our trainees enter residency without any surgical training and leave with both the ability and permission to operate independently.

Richard Bell eloquently outlined some of the modern challenges in surgical education in his well-known article, "Why Johnny cannot operate."[1] He argued that operative skills are acquired and are not innate, and that the current level of experience in operative training is insufficient to achieve competence, let alone proficiency or mastery. He demonstrated that the mean number of procedures performed by graduating general surgical residents was 1022 in 2005. One of the most compelling arguments is made from a bar graph sequentially plotting procedures performed in training with decreasing frequency, beginning with the most commonly performed procedure, laparoscopic cholecystectomy, on the far left, and then in descending order of frequency to the right. Although the average graduate performs more than 300 types of procedures during training, it is evident from this graph that most graduates perform only 18 procedures more than 10 times.[1]

Such calculations have not been made in otolaryngology training, but are likely similar. In otolaryngology—head and neck surgery, we have enjoyed a broadening of our specialty over the past 30 years. This expansion has come at a time when technological advances have allowed for more types of surgical procedures within each domain. Our particular challenge in training to competency in otolaryngology is the diversity of surgical procedures, constrained training time owing to duty-hour requirements, and increased emphasis on supervision and operative efficiency. Together, these factors reduce resident autonomy and limit exposure to core surgical procedures. Countermeasures for consideration include extending the duration of surgical training or shifting surgical teaching outside of the operating theater.

THE COST OF TEACHING IN THE OPERATING ROOM

What is the economic cost of training a surgeon? The modest salary and benefits package is only a small component of the true cost to the training institution. It is probable that we, as surgical educators, significantly underestimate the true costs. Calhoon and colleagues[2] addressed this question by sending cost analysis templates to program directors of 6 thoracic surgery residency programs. Based on the templates, the average annual estimated cost for training was $250,000 per resident. However, when formal accounting evaluations were performed, the annual calculated cost increased to $483,000 per resident, with a range from $330,000 to $667,000.

These cost estimates for residency training do not fully account for the increased cost of OR time related to the involvement of a resident surgeon in a procedure. It has been argued that the increased time required to train surgeons does not increase the cost for the hospital directly, but rather is primarily a "cost" to the attending surgeon, as missed opportunity cost for performing more operative procedures during the same amount of time.[3] However, several studies have demonstrated significant added costs related to surgical trainee involvement.

In plastic surgery, the cost of intraoperative education was estimated by Sasor and colleagues[4] in 2013. They reviewed a single surgeon's experience for cleft lip and cleft palate repair to assess operative time for cases performed with or without a plastic surgery resident or craniofacial fellow. Cases with resident involvement (>85% of cases) averaged 60% to 65% more time than cases without a trainee. Craniofacial fellows, who were likely to have more independence, averaged more than twice the duration as attending surgeon experience alone. This translated to estimated increased costs per case of $275 and $440 for residents and fellows, respectively.[4]

In pediatric otolaryngology, resident participation has been shown to contribute to increased procedure time for common otolaryngology procedures. Puram and colleagues[5] reviewed 3922 procedures and demonstrated that residents had an increased total OR time that ranged from 4.9 minutes (bilateral tympanostomy tubes) to 12.8 minutes (tonsillectomy and adenoidectomy), depending on the duration of the procedure. On average, increases in duration of procedures ranged from 45.6% to 76.1%.

In 2016, Allen and colleagues[6] reviewed 29,134 cases where only 1 Current Procedural Terminology code was entered out of a total of 84,997 cases reviewed. Of the 246 types of procedures reviewed, 45 procedures took significantly longer with a resident present in the room, averaging 4.8 minutes longer. This seems somewhat negligible, but at conservative estimated cost of nearly $10 per minute of operative time, this translated to nearly $500,000 per year of additional cost for the hospital system.

Using this cost analysis as a model, it may be a conservative cost estimate to place the additional cost to a hospital system of a resident procedure at approximately $50 per procedure. When considering that a majority of otolaryngology trainees perform between 1500 and 2000 surgical procedures during their residency, not including procedures as assistant surgeons, the additional cost to the system of resident involvement in surgical procedures may exceed $100,000 per resident in training, simply in additional OR time. For a training program in a large academic center, with multiple residents and fellows per year, these hidden costs begin to mount.

Other hidden costs of training surgeons in the OR include surgical complications and additional morbidity from prolonged anesthesia. A surgical complication may require additional therapy, prolong hospitalization, and incur legal costs. Surgeries that extend beyond regular work hours increase labor costs (overtime) and have an opportunity cost for the surgeon and the hospital.

Surgical educators and hospital administrators interested in cost-savings programs may wish to explore creative ways to implement simulation in a surgical training curriculum. Even modest use of simulation, such as a "warm-up" to surgical procedures, may improve OR performance and efficiency for surgical trainees.[7] Given the yearly expense of surgical training, efforts to reduce the duration of surgical training by using competency-based instead of time-based outcome measures may result in tremendous cost savings to the system (**Table 1**).

WHAT IS IT GOING TO COST?

Although some form of simulation has existed for decades in surgical training, we are truly in the infancy stages of incorporating simulation into residency education. Beginning in July 2008, the Accreditation Council for Graduate Medical Education

Table 1	
Cost differences in learning environments for surgical education	
Learning Environment	**Costs ($/min)**
Operating room	10–183[6,8]
Simulation laboratory	3.30[9]

(ACGME) Residency Review Committee for Surgery mandated that all surgery residency programs incorporate simulation within the curriculum of their program (**Table 2**).

Including physician time, laboratory support, and materials, the total cost for implementing a curriculum for simulation in general surgery based on the American College of Surgeons/Association of Program Directors in Surgery Skulls Curriculum, was estimated at $22,106 by Pentiak and colleagues.[10] Nearly 36% of the cost of the simulation program was attributable to physician salary and time. Calhoon and colleagues[2] described a cost-neutral response to this by redirecting faculty educational time away from already existing nonsimulation education, such as didactic teaching, to simulation.

Like many surgical fields, neurosurgery training in the United States has been significantly affected by ACGME work hour regulations. For this reason, neurosurgery educators have increasingly been using simulation as an adjunct to traditional teaching methods. Gasco and colleagues[8] estimated the per hour cost of simulation in neurosurgery to be approximately $200 per hour. This was significantly lower than the per hour cost estimate for the OR for neurosurgical procedures, which was estimated to range from $2300 to $5500 for the first 30 minutes and $926 to $2756 for each subsequent 30-minute interval.[8] Using this estimate, reducing the operative time by just 10% (6 minutes) would save more than $230 in the first half hour and $92.60 in each subsequent half hour. It is clear from such figures that, for each hour of a case, a few minutes per hour of saved time could fund an entire hour of surgical simulation.

The standardization of fundamentals of laparoscopic surgery has allowed for several studies evaluating the cost and efficiency of simulator training in laparoscopic surgery. Raque and colleagues[9] studied the educational expense of simulator training in a group of 19 surgical residents. The average per resident cost of training using a $5700 simulator over 6 years averaged to $715 per resident. Taking into account the number of cases needed to achieve proficiency (90% of the maximum assessment score), the cost of surgical simulation ranged from nearly $36 to $39 dollars per case. Because simulation training did not shift the learning curve to allow for proficiency to be reached in a fewer number of cases, the authors concluded that simulator experience increased costs without accelerating the learning curve. However, the authors did not account for the cost of saved OR time by shifting the location of the learning outside of the OR. Additionally, the study used an expensive, high-fidelity simulator.[9]

The ACGME is beginning to explore competency-based surgical education as compared with the traditional time-based surgical training models, based on preliminary reports of success from other countries, including Canada. Implementing such a program would require a significant investment in surgical simulation.

So, what is the cost of an all-in approach to surgical simulation training? Nousiainen and colleagues[11] examined the cost of simulation training in orthopedic residency in

Table 2		
Estimated costs of various methods for surgical simulation training		
Simulator Type	**Relative Costs**	**Fidelity**
Task trainer	Low	Low
Ex vivo animal models	Low	Medium
Live animal model	Medium	Medium to high
Human cadaver	Medium	High
Computer-based simulation	Medium to high	Variable

Toronto. At the University of Toronto, a competency-based curriculum has been initiated that relies heavily on simulation. When reviewing all direct financial cost of surgical materials, cadavers, standardized patient costs, artificial models, and faculty time were estimated to be $158,050 USD.[11]

One has to consider not only the cost of the equipment, space, and personnel (faculty and laboratory), but also the downstream costs related to removing residents from the clinical environment. Adding additional time for simulation increases the education to service ratio. Costs for hiring additional full-time equivalent support staff should be considered.[8]

COST CONTAINMENT: SIMULATION ON THE CHEAP

The most realistic, high-fidelity model remains the human cadaver. Cadaver costs fall into a modest price range, relative to other high-fidelity synthetic models. For example, Carey and colleagues[12] describe a low-cost method for perfusing fresh human models by cannulating the femoral vessels and using a perfusion pump. Additionally, mechanical ventilation can be performed with an endotracheal tube and ventilator. The authors advocate that fresh, perfused models replicate human tissue handling and vascular anatomy for surgical dissection. In this study, the perfused model costs averaged $1263 per model.[12] Although this cost is high, multiple surgical specialties may be able to use the same cadaveric model. In otolaryngology, such a model may have a role in head and neck surgeries where vessel volume and pressure are a key component to surgical dissection.

When considering the cost of simulation, task trainers may provide an economically viable alternative to high-fidelity and high-cost models. A low-cost aortic anastomosis model ($22.50/unit) has been demonstrated to improve aortic anastomosis in medical students and residents, with pretest and posttest skills performed on a high-fidelity model.[13] Such studies may provide an archetype for simulation training that can even be used at home.

Such task trainers may indeed be more effective than high-fidelity models. Many task trainers in surgical education have been described, the most recognized and tested of which has been the fundamentals of laparoscopic surgery curriculum. Surgical educators from Winnipeg, Manitoba, compared low-fidelity (fundamentals of laparoscopic surgery) and high-fidelity (LapVR) simulators for surgical training. Although this was a small study of 26 participants, there was improved construct validity and predictive validity with the lower fidelity model when participants were tested intraoperatively performing a human cholecystectomy.[14]

Hernández-Irizarry and colleagues[15] demonstrated that part task training was more effective than whole task training for laparoscopic inguinal hernia repairs. For the 44 general surgery trainees studied, trainees randomized to part task training achieved mastery 17 minutes faster, used fewer materials, and had improved retention of mastery in long-term (1-month) posttesting.

Within the field of otolaryngology, creative, low-cost task trainers have been demonstrated using low cost materials, such as syringes for tympanostomy tube training,[16] chicken wings for endoscopic skull base surgery training,[17] and PVC pipes for nasolaryngoscopy practice,[18] among others. For health care systems without a simulation laboratory, portable, inflatable OR theater enclosures have been described to create an immersive OR environment without the cost of a permanent laboratory space.[19]

COST SAVINGS FROM PREVENTION OF MEDICAL ERRORS

In their *New England Journal of Medicine* article from 2013, Birkmeyer and colleagues[20] demonstrated an association between surgeon technical skills and patient outcomes. Among 20 bariatric surgeons in Michigan who participated in a statewide collaborative improvement project, those in the highest quartile for technical skills by videorating assessment of real surgeries, had a lower risk-adjusted complication rate, were less likely to have cases that required reoperation or readmission, and had shorter operative times.[20] Thus, it seems that competency should not be the standard, but rather mastery. Current residency and fellowship training may not be adequate to achieve mastery and there may be a role for surgical simulation beyond formal training. This role may be especially important as new surgical procedures and technologies are introduced and surgeons strive to acquire new surgical skills.

This concept of continued surgeon coaching with live or video assessment is rare among surgeons, but is highlighted by Atul Gawande in his book *Better: A Surgeon's Notes on Performance* as a possible means to continue to improve throughout the years of posttraining practice.[21] Because the majority of the physician workforce is not currently in training, the benefits of simulation, and therefore the potential cost savings, should not be limited to the time of residency or fellowship. Health systems interested in significant financial savings should strongly consider investing in strategies to improve surgeon technical skills and the efficiency of surgical teams. Until now, the burden has been on the surgeon to seek out and fund such endeavors, but there are clear cost-saving implications for hospital systems. Simulation may also serve as a means for hospital systems to measure surgeon performance more objectively to potentially identify surgeons who would be predicted to have higher risk-adjusted complication rates for particular procedures and to provide targeted programs for skill improvement.

Errors in surgery are common, but many are preventable. Shah and colleagues[22] demonstrated that, among otolaryngologists in practice who responded to a survey from the American Academy of Otolaryngology—Head & Neck Surgery, 66% reported an adverse event within the past 6 months. Using simulation to reduce the errors in operative technique and improve communication between team members may translate to improved medical outcomes and reduced expenditures related to costly complications, reoperations, or medical malpractice claims.

In addition to increasing patient morbidity and mortality, surgical errors are financially costly. The classic report from the Institute of Medicine report "To Err is Human" estimated that between 44,000 and 98,000 deaths occur each year as a result of medical errors, with an estimated $17 billion to $29 billion of costs attributable to preventable adverse events.[23] Specifically for surgery, Encinosa and Hellinger[24] estimated that each error increased 90-day expenditures by as much as $646 to $28,218. Many of these costs (20%) occurred after discharge from the hospital.

The Institute of Medicine report compared the staggering estimate of preventable deaths (up to 98,000) to the number of deaths in US airline fatalities experienced in that same year, namely, zero.[23] There is thus ample evidence to fund large-scale simulation efforts aimed at improving operative performance and decreasing medical errors, as has been accomplished in the airline industry and other high-risk industries in the United States to reduce morbidity, mortality, and their resulting costs.

The idea of an insurance company or hospital system investing heavily in simulation to reduce the risk of future complications seems like an optimist's futuristic dream. However, it is already occurring. The Risk Management Foundation of the Harvard Medical Institutions convened leaders from affiliated institutions and provided financial support to develop a standardized OR team training simulation program.[25] Surgeon participation was incentivized by a 10% reduction in malpractice premiums for participation in the course (approximately $4500 of savings) and continuing medical education credit. The pilot included 221 participants from surgical, anesthesia, and nursing teams, with very positive feedback from participants.

BOTTOM LINE: WHO WILL FOOT THE BILL?

As we have explored, there may be an opportunity for hospital systems, malpractice insurance companies, and even health insurance companies to invest heavily in surgical simulation, because all of these entities have the potential for financial savings by increasing the technical skills of surgeons and improving communication of surgical teams. Until this occurs, departments may consider using current funds earmarked for didactic purposes and redirecting them to simulation education. Incentives could be given for faculty who convert traditional didactic activities to simulation-based interactive sessions.

Industry may be another avenue of support. Already, there is significant industry support for otolaryngology education, for the development of simulation laboratories, "in-kind" donation of industry products for simulation, and industry-supported educational opportunities. But educators and residents must be conscious of and properly disclose these industry relationships. Increasing funding from philanthropic sources or grant funding may minimize such reliance on industry support.

CHALLENGES AND OPPORTUNITIES

One of the most significant challenges to otolaryngology simulation is related to the economy of scale. We are a relatively small specialty. As demonstrated, the per-person cost of simulation education should be expected to decrease with increased numbers of participants. Otolaryngologists have traditionally overcome these barriers by partnering with other institutions to host regional simulation programs.

Continued multiinstitutional collaboration is needed to further the role of simulation within otolaryngology training. Hospitals and insurance companies need to be educated regarding the economic benefits of surgical simulation by professional societies and patient advocacy groups. Further research will better define the visible and hidden costs of the current training paradigm and demonstrate a viable business model for surgical simulation.

Using an analogy put forth by Steve Kaplan in his book, "Bag the Elephant! How to Win and Keep BIG Customers,"[26] we, as surgical educators, must work together to "Bag the Elephant!" and fund surgical simulation.

REFERENCES

1. Bell RH. Why Johnny cannot operate. Surgery 2009;146(4):533–42.
2. Calhoon JH, Baisden C, Holler B, et al. Thoracic surgical resident education: a costly endeavor. Ann Thorac Surg 2014;98(6):2012–5.
3. Babineau TJ, Becker J, Gibbons G, et al. The cost of operative training for surgical residents. Arch Surg 2004;139(4):366–70.
4. Sasor SE, Flores RL, Wooden WA, et al. The cost of intraoperative plastic surgery education. J Surg Educ 2013;70(5):655–9.
5. Puram SV, Kozin ED, Sethi R, et al. Impact of resident surgeons on procedure length based on common pediatric otolaryngology cases. Laryngoscope 2015; 125(4):991–7.
6. Allen RW, Pruitt M, Taaffe KM. Effect of resident involvement on operative time and operating room staffing costs. J Surg Educ 2016;73(6):979–85.
7. Do AT, Cabbad MF, Kerr A, et al. A warm-up laparoscopic exercise improves the subsequent laparoscopic performance of ob-gyn residents- a low-cost laparoscopic trainer. JSLS 2006;10(3):297–301.

8. Gasco J, Holbrook TJ, Patel A, et al. Neurosurgery simulation in residency training: feasibility, cost, and educational benefit. Neurosurgery 2013;73:S39–45.

9. Raque J, Goble A, Jones VM, et al. The relationship of endoscopic proficiency to educational expense for virtual reality simulator training amongst surgical trainees. Am Surg 2015;81(7):747–52.

10. Pentiak PA, Schuch-Miller D, Streetman RT, et al. Barriers to adoption of the surgical resident skills curriculum of the American College of Surgeons/Association of Program Directors in Surgery. Surgery 2013;154(1):23–8.

11. Nousiainen MT, McQueen SA, Ferguson P, et al. Simulation for teaching orthopaedic residents in a competency-based curriculum: do the benefits justify the increased costs? Clin Orthop Relat Res 2016;474(4):935–44.

12. Carey JN, Minneti M, Leland HA, et al. Perfused fresh cadavers: method for application to surgical simulation. Am J Surg 2015;210(1):179–87.

13. Helder MR, Rowse PG, Ruparel RK, et al. Basic cardiac surgery skills on sale for $22.50: an aortic anastomosis simulation curriculum. Ann Thorac Surg 2016; 101(1):316–22.

14. Steigerwald SN, Park J, Hardy KM, et al. Does laparoscopic simulation predict intraoperative performance? A comparison between the fundamentals of laparoscopic surgery and LapVR evaluation metrics. Am J Surg 2015;209(1):34–9.

15. Hernández-Irizarry R, Zendejas B, Ali SM, et al. Optimizing training cost-effectiveness of simulation-based laparoscopic inguinal hernia repairs. Am J Surg 2016;211(2):326–35.

16. Malekzadeh S, Hanna G, Wilson B, et al. A model for training and evaluation of myringotomy and tube placement skills. Laryngoscope 2011;121(7):1410–5.

17. Kaplan DJ, Vaz-Guimaraes F, Fernandez-Miranda JC, et al. Validation of a chicken wing training model for endoscopic microsurgical dissection. Laryngoscope 2015;125(3):571–6.

18. Johnston DI, Selimi V, Chang A, et al. A low-cost alternative for nasolaryngoscopy simulation training equipment: a randomised controlled trial. J Laryngol Otol 2015;129(11):1101–7.

19. Kassab E, Tun JK, Arora S, et al. "Blowing up the barriers" in surgical training: exploring and validating the concept of distributed simulation. Ann Surg 2011; 254(6):1059–65.

20. Birkmeyer JD, Finks JF, O'Reilly A, et al. Surgical skill and complication rates after bariatric surgery. N Engl J Med 2013;369(15):1434–42.

21. Gawande A. Better: a surgeon's notes on performance. 1st edition. New York: Picador; 2008.

22. Shah RK, Boss EF, Brereton J, et al. Errors in otolaryngology revisited. Otolaryngol Head Neck Surg 2014;150(5):779–84.

23. Kohn LT, Corrigan J, Donaldson MS. To err is human: Building a safer health system. Washington, DC: National Academy Press; 2000.

24. Encinosa WE, Hellinger FJ. The impact of medical errors on ninety-day costs and outcomes: an examination of surgical patients. Health Serv Res 2008;43(6): 2067–85.

25. Arriaga AF, Gawande AA, Raemer DB, et al. Pilot testing of a model for insurer-driven, large-scale multicenter simulation training for operating room teams. Ann Surg 2014;259(3):403–10.

26. Kaplan S. Bag the Elephant: How to Win and Keep BIG Customers. New York: Workman; 2008.

Moving?

Make sure your subscription moves with you!

To notify us of your new address, find your **Clinics Account Number** (located on your mailing label above your name), and contact customer service at:

Email: journalscustomerservice-usa@elsevier.com

800-654-2452 (subscribers in the U.S. & Canada)
314-447-8871 (subscribers outside of the U.S. & Canada)

Fax number: 314-447-8029

Elsevier Health Sciences Division
Subscription Customer Service
3251 Riverport Lane
Maryland Heights, MO 63043

*To ensure uninterrupted delivery of your subscription, please notify us at least 4 weeks in advance of move.